Achieving High Quality Care

Practical Experience from NICE

Achieving High Quality Care

Practical Experience from NICE

EDITED BY

Gillian Leng CBE, MBChB, MD, FFPH, FRCP, FRCPEd

Deputy Chief Executive, National Institute for Health and Care Excellence, London, UK;
Visiting Professor, King's College London,
Division of Health and Social Research,
London, UK

Val Moore MFPH, MSc, PGCert Ed

Implementation Programme Director,
National Institute for Health and Care Excellence,
London, UK

Sasha Abraham MRCGP, MBBS, DRCOG, DFSRH

General Practitioner, Tower Hamlets,
London, UK

WILEY Blackwell

This edition first published 2014 © 2014 by John Wiley & Sons, Ltd.

Registered office: John Wiley & Sons, Ltd, The Atrium, Southern Gate, Chichester, West Sussex, PO19 8SQ, UK

Editorial offices: 9600 Garsington Road, Oxford, OX4 2DQ, UK
The Atrium, Southern Gate, Chichester, West Sussex, PO19 8SQ, UK
111 River Street, Hoboken, NJ 07030-5774, USA

For details of our global editorial offices, for customer services and for information about how to apply for permission to reuse the copyright material in this book please see our website at www.wiley.com/wiley-blackwell

Library of Congress Cataloging-in-Publication Data

Achieving high quality care : practical experience from NICE / edited by Gillian Leng, Val Moore, Sasha Abraham.
    p. ; cm.
  Includes bibliographical references and index.
  ISBN 978-1-118-54360-3 (pbk.)
  I. Leng, Gillian, 1960- editor. II. Moore, Val, 1962- editor. III. Abraham, Sasha, editor.
  [DNLM: 1. National Institute for Health and Care Excellence (Great Britain) 2. Quality of Health Care–standards–Great Britain. 3. Patient-Centered Care–methods–Great Britain. 4. Quality Assurance, Health Care–methods–Great Britain. W 84.4 FA1]
  RA395.G6
  362.10941 – dc23

                                                                              2014014237

A catalogue record for this book is available from the British Library.

Wiley also publishes its books in a variety of electronic formats. Some content that appears in print may not be available in electronic books.

Cover image: Courtesy of NICE

Typeset in 9/12pt Palatino by Laserwords Private Limited, Chennai, India
Printed in Singapore by C.O.S. Printers Pte Ltd

1 2014

Contents

List of Contributors

Sasha Abraham
Tower Hamlets, London, UK

Nick Baillie
Indicators, Health and Social Care Quality Team, National Institute for Health and Care Excellence, Manchester, UK

Paul Chrisp
Medicines and Prescribing Centre, National Institute for Health and Care Excellence, Manchester, UK

Jennifer Field
Health Education England, Leeds, UK

Danny Keenan
Manchester Royal Infirmary, Manchester, UK
University of Manchester, Manchester, UK
Department of Cardiothoracic Surgery. Manchester Heart Centre, Central Manchester University Hospitals NHS Foundation Trust, Manchester, UK

Gillian Leng
National Institute for Health and Care Excellence, London, UK
Division of Health and Social Research, King's College London, London, UK

Val Moore
National Institute for Health and Care Excellence, London, UK

Julie Royce
Implementation Support, National Institute for Health and Care Excellence, London, UK

Sara Twaddle
Scottish Intercollegiate Guidelines Network (SIGN), Healthcare Improvement Scotland, Edinburgh, UK

Elaine Whitby
Education & Support, National Institute for Health and Care Excellence, Manchester, UK

Foreword

These are challenging times for everyone working in health care. In every country across the world, the demands and need for care far outstrip the resources available. The complexity of caring for an ageing population with multiple morbidities, the advances of the pharmaceutical industry and the aspirations of clinicians pose real challenges for all the caring professions.

And the phrase 'caring profession' is much more than a cliché. It is a description. Clinicians care. They want to deliver. They want to do the best for their patients. They aspire to real quality, real care.

Since 1999, NICE – an acronym that now stands for the National Institute for Health and Care Excellence – has been producing work that is designed to support every clinician in their aspirations towards quality. NICE's clinical guidelines exist to provide ready access to a comprehensive summary of the best available evidence for quality care, and is developed using international standards for guideline development, which includes a thorough assessment of the literature informed by the views of both patients and clinicians.

But the simple existence of guidelines is not enough, any more than owning a dictionary makes one a writer. Turning guidance into practice can be more than a little challenging, a reality that this book is designed to address. Our patients need and deserve the best care, and this book aims to improve care by helping clinicians use the very best available evidence. Using a deliberately practical approach, which uses numerous examples from everyday care, it covers every facet of quality – whether organisational, theoretical, financial, motivational or practical.

As this book makes clear, the most common factors reported as preventing effective uptake are a lack of clinical leadership and engagement and a lack of resources – and while finances are going to be tight for many years to come, NICE's implementation advice can offer transferable practical support.

And at a time of financial stringency, the use of evidence has to be a vital protection against waste. We owe it to our patients, and we owe it to the National Health Service (NHS), to use evidence, rather than simply go on doing what we have always done just because we have always done it.

Everyone who aspires to improve quality will get real benefit from this book. More importantly, if we use the evidence and we aim for real evidence-based quality, every patient will get real benefit too. What more can we ask for?

Professor David Haslam, CBE
FRCGP, FRCP, FFPH, FAcadMed
Chairman, National Institute for Health and Care Excellence

Preface

When the National Institute for Health and Care Excellence (NICE) was first established in 1999, it was not expecting to play an active role in putting its guidance into practice. It rapidly became clear, however, that encouraging a change in practice at a national level represented a significant challenge, and that NICE needed to take an active role in supporting the implementation of its guidance.

In doing this, over the years we have drawn on a broad range of relevant research evidence, taken advice from experts and listened to those actively involved in generating change. We have analysed various sources of data to give us a picture of the barriers to change and, wherever possible, we have used routine data to track improvements. We have liaised with other national agencies to ensure, as far as possible, that routine systems encourage and support change through mechanisms such as financial incentives and educational initiatives. Ultimately, however, change results from the actions of individuals, and individuals will be most effective when working in a supportive environment.

All of us who have tried to improve health care will know that, however great the benefits of implementing change, making that change happen is not easy. This inevitability was summed up in the sixteenth century by the theologian, Richard Hooker, who said: 'Change is not made without inconvenience, even from worse to better'. The status quo is, by definition, the easiest position to maintain, and changing that position takes energy and drive. In all environments and situations, we must protect enough time and resources to enable individuals to develop new ways of working and to implement effective practice and improve care for patients.

We hope that the practical advice provided in this book will help remind all those working in the health care system of the activities associated with driving forward change.

Gillian Leng, Val Moore, Sasha Abraham
2014

Acknowledgements

We are grateful to the following for their helpful input to the development of this book and for contributing a range of insightful case studies: Nigel Beasley and Owen Bennett, Nicola Bent, Emer Corbett, Paresh Dawda, Shonagh D'Sylva, Liz Eccles, Martin Eccles, Louise Fitzgerald, Matt Fogarty, Robbie Foy, Pamela Griffiths, David Haslam, Rebecca Kearney, Fergus Macbeth, Jane Moore, Maxine Power, Rajini Ramana, Aggie Rawlings, John Sampson, Preeti Sud, Fiona Sutherland, Victoria Thomas and Abigail Warren.

Acknowledgements

Introduction

Gillian Leng[1,2]

[1]*National Institute for Health and Care Excellence, London, UK*
[2]*Division of Health and Social Research, King's College, London, UK*

Introduction

Taking research evidence, interpreting it with input from patients and experts to generate best practice guidance is not straightforward. It is, however, relatively easy compared with the challenges of putting guidance into practice.

The National Institute for Health and Care Excellence (NICE) is very sensitive to this challenge as, since it was first established in 1999, over 900 individual pieces of NICE guidance have been published. These cover a range of topic areas, including the appraisal of new drugs, assessment of new diagnostic tests and other medical technologies, development of clinical guidelines and guidance for public health.

We know that simple dissemination of this best practice guidance is insufficient on its own to generate a change in practice. Indeed, this process could have almost no impact if the guidance is not seen to come from a credible, respected source. Evidence from the implementation literature indicates that no method for getting evidence into practice is effective, and that, to generate any change, efforts are required at national, organisational and individual levels.

The aim of this book is, at a very basic level, simply to help improve patient care through evidence-based practice. It takes a practical approach, starting with an overview of potential systems and processes for those providing health care, followed by more details on how to recognise high-quality guidance. This book then outlines some of the most frequently encountered challenges in changing practice, and suggests practical actions and financial mechanisms that might help overcome some of these challenges. Throughout the book, there are

Achieving High Quality Care: Practical Experience from NICE, First Edition.
Edited by Gillian Leng, Val Moore and Sasha Abraham.
© 2014 John Wiley & Sons, Ltd. Published 2014 by John Wiley & Sons, Ltd.

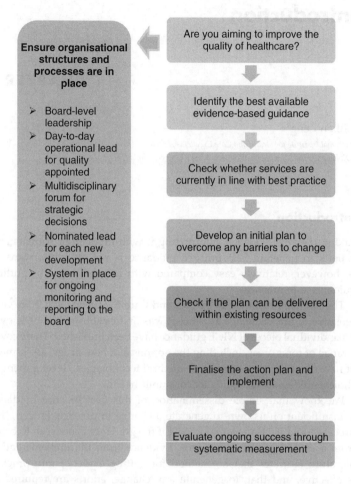

Fig. 1.1 Overview of process for achieving high-quality care.

examples drawn from practice across the National Health Service (NHS), helping to bring to life some of the theoretical concepts.

Figure 1.1 shows the scope of this book, with each chapter expanding on a key part of the whole implementation process necessary to achieve high-quality care.

What is the role of evidence?

The development of 'evidence-based medicine' as the underpinning approach to inform clinical practice is the approach that has grown and developed over a period of about 50 years. The history of using experimentation to confirm the effects of treatment goes back much further – one of the earliest clinical trials was conducted in 1747 by James Lind. He compared the effects of various acidic substances on sailors with scurvy and demonstrated that those given citrus fruits recovered after 6 days [1].

An expansion in the numbers of randomised controlled trials occurred rapidly in the 1950s and 1960s, increasing the body of evidence available to practitioners. This prompted Archie Cochrane to write critically about the lack of any systematic collection of research evidence in his 1972 publication, *Effectiveness and Efficiency* [2]. His criticisms spurred new, rigorous evaluations of health care interventions, and eventually led to the development of the Cochrane Collaboration in 1991.

There is no doubt that the methodology behind the rigorous development of systematic reviews has contributed greatly to an advance in medical knowledge. The research evidence base is seldom complete, however, as eloquently described by Lomas and colleagues: 'Evidence is inherently uncertain, dynamic, complex, contestable and rarely complete' [3]. This statement is illustrated in areas of medicine such as prognosis and diagnosis where there is relatively little research, and by the frequent absence of elderly patients with complex medical problems from randomised controlled trials.

The development of clinical guidelines provides a methodology to help overcome some of the issues generated by the variability in research evidence. Using a group process that facilitates input from relevant patients and experts, it is possible to generate a set of practical recommendations for practitioners informed by the best available evidence. This sometimes entails an extrapolation of the evidence, but the process also highlights gaps in the evidence with the aim of stimulating future research to answer key questions. The most sophisticated clinical guidelines, such as those developed by NICE, also incorporate an economic analysis alongside a review of the evidence on effectiveness.

A robust clinical guideline, therefore, represents a synthesis of the best available evidence, which has been interpreted by clinicians and patients to generate a set of practical recommendations. These recommendations, and the way in which they are phrased and presented, become key to stimulating a change in practice. They represent the 'front face' of the evidence, and must be sufficiently clear and concise to communicate the appropriate action required. Further details on the methodology of guideline development and how it helps drive implementation is given in Chapter 3.

How can guidance be used to track improvement?

The case for using guidance to inform clinical practice and improve patient care is a strong one. Assuming that the guidance has been developed using robust methodology, it will represent a statement of best practice informed by a comprehensive review of the evidence. Systematic use of this guidance will, therefore, have the benefits of

- ensuring that all practitioners are providing up-to-date care in line with the evidence;
- increasing standardisation of care across the country;
- improving access to new drugs and technologies that are considered cost effective;
- ensuring that patients benefit by receiving better care and by being informed about the treatments they should expect.

Guidelines represent one of the most important elements of evidence-based practice in health care. Clinicians often use them as stand-alone documents, but the recommendations are increasingly found embedded in electronic decision support systems where the doctor may not even recognise them as guidelines. The importance of using evidence-based guidelines is reinforced by medical defence organisations, which expect any variation in care from best practice guidance to be documented. Variation can of course be entirely appropriate – guidelines are not 'rules' – but it is important that a guideline is always considered, even if the recommendations are not then deemed appropriate in a particular individual.

Guidelines are often long documents, providing a comprehensive set of recommendations for a particular disease or condition. This is important in providing a complete overview of best practice, but can be challenging both in terms of identifying the most important areas for change and for tracking progress towards improvement. To support a focus on areas of improvement, NICE now uses guidance recommendations to generate a prioritised set of 'quality statements', which are concise, measurable statements designed to drive quality improvements across a pathway of care.

The benefits of prioritised quality statements are that they provide:

- a set of priority areas where improvements are most likely to be required;
- concise statements with associated measures and indicators to facilitate measurement of progress;
- a potential mechanism to incentivise improvements;
- a simple focus on high-quality care that is accessible to patients.

Where possible, quality standard statements will be associated with routinely measured indicators, with data collected and collated at a national level. This will greatly ease the burden of data collection at a local level. In other cases, measurement will require local audit, building on the well-recognised tradition of linking audit with guidelines. The benefits of audit in driving a change in practice will be covered later in this book.

What are the challenges to achieving quality improvement?

The concept of quality is a broad one and is generally recognised to mean either a statement of best practice (high quality) or a process of continuous quality improvement. A widely accepted description of quality across the NHS is probably the one defined by Lord Darzi in *High Quality Care for All* [4]. It describes a process of continuous quality improvement encompassing three elements: patient safety, clinical effectiveness and patient experience. NICE takes into account these three elements in producing guidance and setting associated quality measures. Sometimes, this description of high-quality care set out by NICE is aspirational and requires significant change to achieve.

There is no comprehensive mechanism, at a national level in England, for routinely tracking successful improvements that result from the adoption of NICE guidance recommendations. Wherever possible, NICE works with other organisations to gather as complete a picture of adoption as possible. This includes where NICE recommendations have been used in national audits and the analysis of routinely collected data that provides a proxy measure of impact.

In some cases, feedback demonstrates that new guidance has a rapid impact on practice such as in the prescribing of a new drug. In other areas, impact is much slower and, anecdotally, the reasons for this are often reported to be a lack of clinical leadership, a lack of money and poor support from health care managers.

To provide a more systematic picture of the challenges encountered when trying to implement NICE guidance, a survey of health care clinicians and managers was commissioned to obtain their views on the most important issues. Responses were received from 683 individuals, of which 41% reported that the most important barrier was gaining consensus with colleagues (Figure 1.2). This resonates with the informal feedback about lack of clinical leadership being an important barrier to change.

The survey showed that lack of money was considered relatively unimportant in influencing adoption (14% of respondents), although two of the other highlighted issues (requirements for new equipment and for training) are also associated with a need for resources. Taken together, these

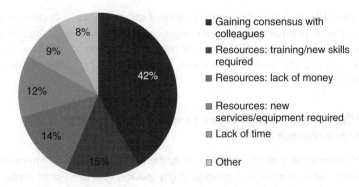

Fig. 1.2 Challenges of implementing NICE guidance – results from a survey of 683 clinicians and managers in 2011.

three factors represent 41% of the total. The remaining factors affecting the implementation of any particular piece of guidance will vary, but this survey illustrates an overview associated with recommendations from NICE.

When health care systems are under pressure financially, the adoption of quality improvement initiatives is likely to become even more challenging. There is a perception that quality improvement and achieving financial balance sit at opposite ends of the spectrum. How financial challenges and other challenges can be systematically overcome to put guidance into practice are addressed later in this book.

How does NICE support implementation?

There are many well-recognised approaches to generating quality improvements such as Six Sigma, Lean and PDSA (Plan, Do, Study, Act). These are often used very successfully at a local level to support the uptake of NICE guidance. NICE's implementation strategy sits alongside these mechanisms and is based on evidence of effective change and informed by feedback from end-users. It is practically focused and designed to build on the evidence-based guidance and provide support for those using it at a local level.

The NICE implementation strategy has four key elements:
• raising awareness of the need to change;
• motivating and inspiring people to change;
• providing practical support to facilitate change;
• evaluating and monitoring the impact of the strategy.

These elements are very much designed to support clinicians and managers to take forward change themselves, as local ownership is essential.

The strategy, therefore, places significant emphasis on influencing external and organisational factors that will stimulate local leadership.

Raising awareness

Raising awareness of the need to do something differently, for example as highlighted in a guideline, is a crucial first step in changing behaviour. For an organisation such as NICE, this function means having an effective dissemination strategy. NICE therefore aims to provide information directly to a range of audiences, including individual practitioners and those managing and funding health care services. This information is also provided indirectly via third parties such as professional journals and other websites. On the NICE website, all types of NICE guidance have been mapped into an interactive pathway presentation, which makes it much easier and quicker to identify the appropriate recommendations.

Motivating change

This element of the strategy is about encouraging individuals and organisations to recognise the importance of evidence-based guidance, not just because of improved patient care, but also because it will help deliver benefits in other areas. In practice, this means aligning NICE guidance and standards with the strategic objectives of other health care organisations. Examples of where this 'joined up' approach is helpful include:

- incorporating NICE guidance in educational modules, such as those produced by Royal Colleges, linked with CPD (Continuing Professional Development) points for those who complete the modules;
- embedding the cost of NICE recommendations into any relevant national tariffs, as this ensures that there is no financial disincentive to not adopt a new technology;
- aligning recommendations from NICE guidance to the primary care financial incentive system, the Quality and Outcomes Framework, to encourage a change in practice in primary care;
- building recommendations from NICE guidance into any national audits;
- working with charitable organisations that can help ensure information is effectively disseminated to patients. Utilising the enthusiasm and energy of patient organisations to provide onward dissemination of key recommendations provides more capacity than could otherwise be provided by NICE and reaches a greater number of individuals.
- using the enthusiasm of leaders in the field to motivate others. NICE also works with dedicated NICE Fellows and Scholars who receive training about evidence-based practice to act as advocates for change.

Practical support

The practical support provided by NICE aims to make things easier for organisations by providing some of the tools and information they may need to help implement recommendations for best practice. The types of products we produce, and when we produce them, are informed by the published evidence and feedback from stakeholder organisations in relation to a particular topic area. There are more details on the practical, local steps required for change later in the book.

Monitoring impact

A core element of any programme is a process for monitoring impact. This process applies to implementation projects at a local level as well as to national programmes. For NICE, it means obtaining both qualitative feedback on the guidance and support materials, and also generating quantitative data to determine uptake of recommendations from NICE.

Summary overview

In summary, evidence-based guidance should be robust and developed in consultation with clinicians and patients. An effective dissemination mechanism should ensure that it is received by the appropriate audience, but in the majority of cases there are likely to be a number of challenges to putting it into practice. The most common factors reported as preventing effective uptake are a lack of clinical leadership and engagement and a lack of resources. NICE has an implementation strategy, based on the evidence of effective implementation, designed to provide support for local implementers. How these fit into a systematic local approach for implementation is described in the rest of the book.

Learning from practice

1 NICE guidance represents a robust set of evidence-based recommendations, informed by the views of clinicians and patients.
2 An effective dissemination mechanism is an essential first step in changing practice, but this would not be sufficient on its own.
3 Changing practice is likely to require a range of different approaches, and this book will illustrate practical examples of where this has been successful.
4 Ongoing monitoring of progress towards implementation is facilitated by the measures accompanying NICE guidance.

References

1 Lind, J. (1753) *A Treatise of the Scurvy in Three Parts. Containing an inquiry into the Nature, Causes and Cure of that Disease, Together with a Critical and Chronological View of What Has Been Published on the Subject*, A. Millar, London.
2 Cochrane, A. (1972) *Effectiveness and Efficiency. Random Reflections on Health Services*, Nuffield Trust, London.
3 Lomas, J., Culyer, T., McCutcheon, C. *et al.* (2005) *Conceptualizing and Combining Evidence For Health System Guidance*, CHSRF.
4 Darzi A. (2008) High Quality Care for ALL. NHS Next Stage Review Final Report. The Stationery Office, London.

Further reading

Greenhalgh, T., Robert, G., Bate, P. *et al.* (2005) *Diffusion of Innovations in Health Service Organisations: A Systematic Literature Review*, Blackwell BMJ Books, Oxford.
Grol, R. and Grimshaw, J. (2003) From best evidence to best practice: effective implementation of change in patients' care. *Lancet*, **362** (9391), 1225–1230.
Fixsen, D.L., Naoom, S.F., Blasé, K.A. *et al.* (2005) *Implementation Research: A Synthesis of the Literature*, University of South Florida, Louis de la Parte Florida Mental Health Institute, The National Implementation Research Network, Tampa, FL (FMHI Publication # Available from: http://nirn.fmhi.usf.edu/resources/publications/monograph/ accessed 10 April 2014).
Grol, R., Wensing, M. and Eccles, M. (eds) (2013) *Improving Patient Care: The Implementation of Change in Clinical Practice*, Elsevier, Edinburgh.

Example in Practice

Using clinical leaders to improve patient care

A Critical Care Network in the East of England applied NICE guidance to improve the prevention, diagnosis and management of delirium. The network achieved this through a range of measures, such as auditing practice, educating staff and sharing practice on the use of new drug therapies.

'Having staff champion the cause of delirium was an effective way of engaging clinicians'.

Source: Emer Corbett, Service Improvement Lead.

NICE guidance highlights room for improvement

Delirium is a common and serious condition, affecting people in hospital or long-term care. It is characterised by changes in mental state or consciousness, which is often shown as confusion, difficulties with understanding and memory or personality changes.

Up to 80% of patients experience at least one episode of delirium in a critical care unit. The condition is associated with higher 6-month mortality and longer hospital stays in patients receiving mechanical ventilation.

Before the project started, the Critical Care Network had already taken certain measures to tackle delirium across the four hospitals it serves. These included implementing the Richmond Agitation Sedation Scale and the Confusion Assessment Method Intensive Care Unit (CAM ICU) in all units to support the early recognition and treatment of delirium.

However, following the publication of NICE's clinical guideline on delirium in 2010, the network observed that more measures could be taken to improve levels of care for patients in its units.

It consequently set a plan of action to ensure care followed NICE recommendations and for improvements to be made in the services for patients at risk of delirium.

Audit reveals areas where care can be improved

The first measure taken was to carry out a baseline audit of current practice across the four hospitals the network serves, using NICE's audit tool as a template. The audit results were then analysed and the network collaborated with the hospitals to draw up local action plans. The hospitals used NICE's implementation tools to formulate these plans and set short time frames for completion.

Delirium champions were identified in each hospital, and training was provided to staff on various topics such as bedside teaching. The delirium champions also raised the focus of delirium on in-house teaching days.

The delirium champions encouraged daily assessment of patients with delirium, as this can lead to early recognition and treatment of the condition. The network observed that tackling the condition early on can also lead to improved patient experience, and savings within critical care due to a reduction in length of stay.

Further measures included featuring CAM ICU assessment scoring boxes on nursing team handover sheets, hosting a *Delirium Month* and a CPD-accredited conference to maintain awareness and sharing practice on new drug therapies.

Increased compliance with NICE guidance

The network has seen improvements in the diagnosis, in management and in the documenting of patient care, with daily assessment now occurring.

Several improvements have also been seen in compliance with NICE-recommended interventions for the prevention of delirium. These include increasing compliance with NICE guidance from 80% to 100% on providing

- appropriate lighting to address cognitive impairment and/or disorientation among patients and
- appropriate noise levels to promote good sleep patterns.

Challenges met included a lack of interest and some scepticism among clinicians. This was tackled through holding a delirium conference, which from delegate feedback showed that it had a positive effect on engagement.

Learning from practice

- It is important to identify delirium champions early on and build on existing relationships to promote the cause.
- Staff engagement is crucial.
- Education, through events such as conferences and galvanised clinicians, provides an opportunity for networking.
- Peer reviews led to better outcomes and sharing of good practice.

Practical actions for health care providers

CHAPTER 2

Val Moore

National Institute for Health and Care Excellence, London, UK

Introduction

NICE may be the pre-eminent developer of guidance in England and beyond, as described more fully in Chapter 3, but it does not have formal accountability for implementation. NICE does, however, encourage implementation within the wider health system through regulation, priority setting, commissioning and local leadership. Health care provider organisations themselves need to take action to ensure their boards, service delivery teams and staff, and of course patients know what is aspired towards and expected.

Successful implementation of guidance depends on understanding the context and circumstances surrounding its relevance to the organisation, and thinking carefully about the gap between current practice and guidance. Selectively deploying one or more of a number of tailored tools or activities (as described in Chapter 4) will increase the likelihood of success in implementation, whatever the topic area happens to be.

The literature and experience of many, including as reported through the NICE fellows and scholars schemes mentioned in Chapter 1, reflect the fact that health care delivery systems have hierarchies and are of complex organisations. Even the most motivated individuals have to understand how these bureaucracies work as well as acquire the leadership skills required to win the hearts and minds of those around them.

NICE has learned that an organisation that has policies, processes and procedures to support the assimilation of new guidance for its services can greatly help the motivation, efforts and success of the leaders of

Achieving High Quality Care: Practical Experience from NICE, First Edition.
Edited by Gillian Leng, Val Moore and Sasha Abraham.
© 2014 John Wiley & Sons, Ltd. Published 2014 by John Wiley & Sons, Ltd.

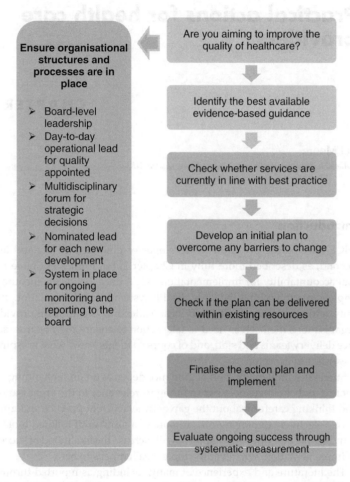

Fig. 2.1 Organisational structures and processes for improving the quality of health care.

change within the many teams delivering treatment and care. This chapter will help those with a formal role in implementation within their local provider organisation. This role may be the day-to-day operational lead for quality or a senior member of the board. If it is more focused on a particular service area, then it may relate more to the role described later as the lead for a new development.

Figure 2.1 shows the overall implementation process with the most relevant aspects for this chapter summarised on the left hand side. More detailed discussion about the actions covered on the right of the flow chart follows in other chapters but is touched upon here in the context of having a good organisational process.

Why take a systematic approach to guidance implementation in a health care provider organisation?

A systematic application of evidence-based guidance, by health care professionals and managers, helps to ensure consistent improvements in people's health outcomes and equal access to processes of care. Chapter 3 illustrates how it is possible to distinguish high-quality evidence-based from other, less robust, guidance. A systematic process also helps to target resources to where they will have the most impact. It can also help to reassure patients, and those who plan and pay for services, if providers of services have a clear process for using high-quality guidance. The following sections show some more specific contextual challenges and benefits for providers of having a systematic approach to handling evidence-based guidance within their organisation.

Legal and regulatory context

Provider organisations need to have regard to any relevant legal requirements, such as those that relate to quality improvement and standards of care, and meet any associated regulatory standards or inspection regimes. The advice in this chapter on the organisational arrangements required to help health care organisations identify and manage relevant guidance to improve care that will fit well with any local management infrastructure to support quality improvement, for example governance, audit departments and other knowledge management functions. These teams and their leaders are pivotal for strategic as well as day-to-day matters on quality.

Cost pressures and quality improvement

The pressure on health care resources put against increasing patient expectations and demand is a pressing problem for all levels of health care. Using accredited guidance (see Chapter 3) may help cut costs while at the same time maintaining and improving service quality. Assessing the potential cost impact of new guidance is a key to local planning (see Chapter 5). A growing collection of quality assured case studies from NICE shows how quality, productivity – and sometimes cash releasing savings – can be achieved through changing service delivery. NICE estimates that if the examples in the collection were adopted by just 50% of eligible organisations in England, they have the potential to save the NHS in England over £2 billion.

Public and patient involvement

Health care professionals want to ensure that they deliver the best possible care they can for their patients. With widespread access to the internet, patients are increasingly asking health professionals about NICE guidance and other sources of patient information. Involving patients in service change is also important for success [1] as is their involvement in guidance development itself.

Staff training and continuing professional development

Training, induction to a new workplace setting and continuing development are the important aspects of professional life. Implementing best practice guidance can provide individuals with assurance about the quality of their own practice, as well as that of the services they offer. NICE provide a continuing professional development function on its website to help professionals or managers capture, annotate and organise information and learning from the information they access on the site. Learning resources for teams or individuals accompany many guidelines and are an increasingly valued part of the NICE implementation portfolio.

What defines quality improvement for health care providers?

Assuming that a systematic approach to quality improvement within a health care organisation is desirable, it is worth stepping back to review how quality in this context has been defined. Definitions of quality vary between and within disciplines, including across the health service. Those who have attempted a definition of quality generally relate it to a statement of what high quality looks like and the quality assurance processes required to achieve it, or to a process of continuous quality improvement [2], or to customer experience.

The actions in Box 2.1 bring together elements of motivation and leadership at the individual and team levels, and the development of action-oriented measurement strategies [3] seen as part of the wider system is discussed further in Chapter 6.

Box 2.1 Eight areas for action to improve health care services

Quality in a service such as health care requires the following eight orientated actions.
- Commitment to excellence for those reliant on the service – excellence judged by those who rely on it as well as technical experts.
- Translation of good ideas into action, often by small incremental persistent steps rather than by large leaps, and always tested against external indicators of performance.
- Emphasis on team rather than individual performance as service depends on a combination of skills, not just on one individual or discipline acting alone.
- Systematic elimination of waste and of barriers to, and flaws in, high performance: excellence may be hard to define, but failures that are remedial can be much more easily identified and acted on.
- Recognition that every job involves responsibility (individual and collective) not only for doing the job well, but for continually finding ways to do it even better.
- Use of concepts (like the six dimensions and measures of performance) diagnostically to determine when and for whom intervention to raise quality is justified and assess the impacts of these interventions.
- Development of action-orientated measurement systems that test progress and hence support continuing improvement.
- Determination to always see quality initiatives in the broader context of quality in the system as a whole. Otherwise, there is a danger that any initiative will be at the expense of an unrecognised loss of quality elsewhere.

Source: Maxwell R. J. Dimensions of quality revisited: from thought to action. Quality Health Care 1992; 1:171–177. Reproduced with permission of the BMJ, London.

Box 2.1 shows how, as well as taking individual and team considerations into account, a focus on the processes by which new ideas and concepts become accepted within an organisation can help an understanding of quality improvement. Knowledge can become implemented, made routine and accepted as routine practice [4]. Processes can facilitate the involvement of key individuals, be stable and predictable, analysed, controlled and improved (such as Lean Six Sigma or the Plan-Do-Study-Act cycle – see Chapter 7). These may be used within a specific area of implementation or applied to an overall organisational approach that is the focus of the practical advice later. Chapter 4 will explore more of the cognitive and behavioural aspects of implementation theory and practice.

What practical advice do health care providers require?

Having taken a broad view of quality improvement, the challenge is now to translate evidence-informed practices into practical advice in an organisational setting. NICE encourages health care providers to continuously improve their services by establishing processes for regularly reviewing their practice against guidance and standards. NICE supports this through the production of specific implementation tools for guidance and by providing general advice on appropriate systems and processes to facilitate guidance uptake. Through direct engagement via the NICE field team (eight consultants working with local organisations) and also through working with other organisations at the national level, NICE has an effective feedback loop that helps it identify what works. This involves listening to, informing and influencing those with a role in improving quality of health care at the local level to share good practice and learning.

Our implementation advice [5] consists of key components as illustrated in Figure 2.1. The NICE website contains more detail on who to involve and for what, the role of a 'NICE manager' combined with other related duties, a process (and microprocesses for particular types of guidance) and pointers to key resources from NICE. The sections that follow are transferable to health care provider organisations in other countries. The development of a new process will always require discussion and buy-in from stakeholders, and local modifications are therefore understandable.

The evidence base and our local experience show that there are several high-level components to a successful implementation process:
• board support and clear leadership;
• day-to-day lead for quality;
• multidisciplinary forum to take strategic decisions;
• nominated lead for each new development;
• a systematic approach to financial planning (details in Chapter 5);
• a systematic approach to implementing guidance (details in Chapter 4);
• a process to evaluate uptake and feedback (details in Chapter 6).

An organisation's approach to meeting these components should be clearly stated in an implementation policy. This should be agreed across the organisation or health community and approved by the boards of the organisations involved. The following sections focus on the first three of the points mentioned earlier and then set the scene for subsequent chapters by introducing the themes of financial planning, implementation and evaluation.

Why board support and clear leadership for achieving high-quality care is important?

Ultimate responsibility for ensuring an organisation is implementing NICE guidance is with the chief executive, but this is often devolved to others, such as the medical director. Directors and senior level stakeholders should receive regular internal reports on the local use of guidance, including audit reports, highlighting areas where the organisation does not provide its services in line with best practice recommendations or there are weaknesses identified in service provision. The risks raised by this should be identified and recorded.

Who should be the day-to-day lead for quality?

Identifying a designated person who will coordinate local quality activities is, in our experience, vital. The responsibilities of this person could include

- coordinating an organisational response to guidance consultations;
- monitoring guidance as it is published and ensuring that they are assessed for relevance to the organisation's services;
- disseminating guidance to key groups and identifying nominated leads to implement the guidance (either within the organisation or by those commissioned to provide the relevant services);
- horizon scanning and informing forward planning, including preparing briefings on the potential impact (including financial impact) of implementing the guidance;
- ensuring an effective documented process for monitoring and feedback is in place and adhered to;
- producing regular senior level reports;
- ensuring that entries are made to the relevant risk register to record deviation from NICE recommendations;
- arranging educational events.

To ensure effective onward dissemination, the day-to-day quality lead could work with others in order to:

- Include information about best practice guidance in induction training for all staff.
- Liaise with the education and training team to access educational forums.
- Link with existing clinical networks, where appropriate. This might include patient's pathway-specific networks, drug and therapeutic committees, and public health networks.

- Develop newsletters, leaflets, prescribing updates or information packs for different audiences.
- Incorporate guidance into local policies and protocols, and ensure that any shared care protocols are updated.

Do you have an effective multidisciplinary forum for strategic decision-making on the use of best practice guidance?

To be most effective, this forum should be a decision-making body that reports to the highest level group in the organisation, typically the board. It could be an existing forum that already serves other functions within the organisation.

The forum should provide overall management, planning and monitoring of implementing guidance. This forum should consider all new guidance shortly after publication, consider their relevance to the organisation and identify named leads and networks to support the implementation of specific guidance recommendations. This multidisciplinary forum should have the following parameters:

- Ensure that effective forward planning and engagement occurs;
- Assess the relevance of new guidance for the organisation as they are published;
- Ensure guidance is disseminated to the appropriate people;
- Identify named leads (see later) to lead on each new development;
- Ensure that the organisation knows its current position regarding all relevant guidance;
- Record deviation from relevant recommendations, and ensure strategies for achieving it in the future are agreed if appropriate;
- Ensure delivery against local action plans;
- Review local audit action plans and results where necessary;
- Check that appropriate financial arrangements are in place (see later).

It is important to consider ways of coordinating work across the health community, especially where guidance covers the primary and secondary care interface, or across health and social care. Collaboration across the community reduces duplication of effort and ensures a coordinated, standardised response to each piece of guidance across the locality. This will help to ensure seamless care.

The case study in Box 2.2 illustrates the process taken to prioritise action by a health care provider organisation in England with respect to NICE guidance.

Box 2.2 Prioritising action on guidance within a health care provider

In 2009, Nottingham University Hospitals Clinical Effectiveness Committee developed new systems and processes for dealing with NICE clinical guidelines. This included identification of a clinical lead for each piece of guidance and asking them to evaluate our compliance against guidance, establishing multidisciplinary task and finish groups, to take action where required.

These groups indicated that it would be impossible to comply with every recommendation owing to the configuration of existing services or the level of investment required to fully comply with each recommendation. To help prioritise areas for development, we asked the clinical leads and their groups to risk assess partial and non-compliance using the trust risk assessment tool and describe the actions required to minimise the risk.

The risk assessment tool evaluates the risk to patients or staff, and the financial and reputation risks to the organisation, grading the risk from low harm to severe harm or death. These scores are multiplied by the likelihood of the risk occurring giving a score between 0 (no risk) and 25 (highest level of risk).

Low-risk non-compliance (0–12) is managed at directorate level, medium risk (13–15) is managed by the trust Clinical Effectiveness Committee and high risk of non-compliance (16–25) is passed up to the Quality Operation Group and Trust Board for action. Risk scores for NICE clinical guidelines are updated and reviewed at the bimonthly Clinical Effectiveness Committee giving the trust a good overview of compliance with NICE guidance and allowing us to prioritise areas for development.

Source: Reproduced with permission of Owen Bennett and Nigel Beasley, Nottingham University Hospitals NHS Trust.

Why a lead for each new development should be nominated?

This role is likely to be a prominent figure that will champion the guidance and inspire others to successful implementation. Often they nominate themselves. If the guidance covers more than one organisation such as primary and secondary care, establish contact with the identified leads in partner organisations to work collaboratively to develop a seamless leadership and action plan.

The person named as the organisational lead for implementing the piece of guidance should work with colleagues to compare current practice with the recommendations. Baseline assessment tools (gap analysis) for clinical guidelines can help organisations to evaluate whether their local practice is generally in line with recommendations before prioritising and embarking on change.

Clinical audit is a quality improvement process that seeks to improve patient care and outcomes by measuring the quality of care against a standard and making improvements where necessary. Organisations may choose to conduct a clinical audit of their current practice against the guidance, in order to make improvements. Re-audit should form part of the audit cycle.

Why take a systematic approach to financial planning for service change?

There is more on this in Chapter 5. The financial implications of implementing any change needs to be an integral part of an organisation's financial and business plans. Preparatory work should begin early, ideally based on draft guidance, and include looking at local services and processes. In some health services, payment for activity or outcomes may nominally include the costs of implementing best practice guidance. In this case, those funding the service will expect providers to deliver accordingly without additional funding. For activity that is outside of such mechanisms, organisations should specify the process for negotiating funding between those who pay and the providers.

Organisations might need to consider capital requirements (equipment), staffing and training requirements, and capacity issues. These will need to be addressed by local delivery and planning processes. You should also consider whether any long-term savings can be made as a result of early actions to promote health and wellbeing. It is important that organisations have a process for working together with local partners to implement NICE guidance as it can help out even the costs and savings.

Developing an action plan

Following a baseline assessment or gap analysis, if services are not in line with best practice guidance, development of an action plan will set out the steps needed to put the guidance into practice. Look at the recommendations that the baseline assessment identified as not currently being carried out, and choose interventions and assign actions to each one. Organisations should assess how much it will cost (or save) to implement the action plan developed following your baseline assessment. It might be possible to make some of the required changes using existing resources, or there may be the potential for savings to be achieved, or capacity freed up to be used for other things. NICE has produced a guide on how to change practice to help health professionals understand, identify and plan to overcome barriers to change [6]. It provides practical suggestions based on evidence on how to identify the barriers to change and select the right method to overcome each one, and includes real-life examples. These issues are covered in Chapter 4.

Once the action plan and assessment of cost have been approved by the relevant group, the work to implement the action plan begins. To enable effective implementation, all partner organisations should sign up to the action plan. It is important to consider ways of coordinating work across the health care community. Collaboration across the community reduces duplication of effort and ensures a coordinated, standardised response to each piece of guidance across the locality.

Evaluate uptake, provide high-level assurance and share your success story

Make sure you evaluate your action plans to analyse how effective they have been and review the impact of the overall implementation process. Regular reporting of progress to the board ensures high-level sign off and provides public transparency, detailing the use of evidence-based guidance into practice. When the process works well, experience shows us that it is important to publicise it. Sharing from success and identifying where further improvement is needed help everyone.

Sustaining improvement and developing and using routine information sources to indicate this is an important legacy of the hard work to initiate change in the first place. This is the focus of Chapter 6.

Summary

This chapter has made the case for taking a systematic approach to guidance implementation in a health care provider organisation. A brief look at definitions of quality has provided background to some practical advice on the roles of key individuals and organisational structures and processes for health care providers.

The scene is set to look in more detail next about the features of guidance that should be looked for in order to inform changes in services with confidence.

Learning from practice

1 The benefits of a systematic approach to using guidance help to address a range of contemporary challenges facing the health care provider.
2 Evidence and experience show that there are seven key practical components to successful implementation within provider organisations.
3 A detailed organisational process and the positive actions of managers and clinical leaders are required to implement change.

References

1 NICE (2008) Community engagement (PH9).
2 Darzi, A. (2008) *High Quality Care for All: NHS Next Stage Review Final Report.* The Stationary Office, London.
3 Maxwell, R.J. (1992 September) Dimensions of quality revisited: from thought to action. *Quality Health Care,* **1** (3), 171–177.
4 Novotna, G., Dobbins, M. & Henderson, J. (2012) Institutionalization of evidence-informed practices in healthcare settings. *Implementation Science,* **7**, 112.
5 NICE (2005) How to put NICE guidance into practice.
6 NICE (2006) How to change practice.

Further reading

Grol, R., Wensing, M., Eccles, M. & Davis, D. (2013) *Improving Patient Care: The Implementation of Change in Health Care,* 2nd edn. Wiley-Blackwell, Chichester.
McMaster University www.healthsystemsevidence.org (accessed 10 April 2014).
NICE Field Team www.nice.org.uk/usingguidance/niceimplementationprogramme (accessed 10 April 2014).
NICE Guidance for the Public www.nice.org.uk/patientsandpublic/index.jsp (accessed 10 April 2014).
NICE Into Practice Website www.nice.org.uk/usingguidance/niceimplementation-tools/howtoguide.

Example in Practice

A hospital-wide approach to reduce mortality among acutely ill patients

A hospital in the South East of England improved the care of its patients by applying recommendations from NICE clinical guidelines on acutely ill patients in hospital.

> We have seen significant reductions in rates for mortality and cardiac arrest since the project started.

Source: Annette Schreiner, Medical Director.

Promptly escalating care for deteriorating patients

A hospital in the South East of England's mortality rates had been higher than average for a number of years, and ONS official figures showed that mortality rates in Dartford had been worse than in any London borough.

To address the mortality issues, the hospital set up a project called *deteriorating patients*. The project's aims were to reduce the hospital's rates of mortality, cardiac arrest and the number of admissions to intensive therapy units (ITUs).

Since 2007, the project has since been continuously evaluated, refined and amended, and has incorporated recommendations from NICE guidance on acutely ill patients in hospital.

Among the key priorities for implementation in this guideline is that hospitals should deliver a graded response strategy for patients identified as being at risk of clinical deterioration. NICE says this strategy should consist of three levels, and a medical team with critical care competencies and diagnostic skills should respond immediately if patients are at high risk of clinical deterioration.

The hospital followed these recommendations to set up a Medical Emergency Team (MET), which helped improve the care of acutely ill patients.

How did the hospital carry out the project?

In 2007, the hospital introduced a patient-at-risk (PAR) scoring system to assess hospital inpatients and provide clinical staff with a measure of level of patients' risk.

This was followed by running ALERT (acute life-threatening events recognition and treatment) training courses for staff to help them recognise patient deterioration and to act appropriately in treating the acutely unwell.

Following this, the hospital started developing the MET, which was subsequently launched in 2008. The MET consists of a medical registrar and an anaesthetic registrar, both of whom are on-call, and an ITU outreach team.

The hospital ensured the team can be contacted via the same system as cardiac arrest teams. The team sees patients, who score the highest risk of deterioration, within 15 minutes of being called out. Patients scoring at less risk will be reviewed by the ward team within the hour, and if the risk score is even less, the patients are reported to the ward sister.

Improving rates for mortality and cardiac arrest

Data from the ITU show that since the project began, patients are being admitted to the unit less unwell, suggesting a timelier response for acutely ill patients. Data for that time also show that ITU mortality has dropped from 21% to 14%.

Results for the whole hospital include the following:

- A 39% reduction of crude mortality rate for all admissions from 2.55% to 1.55%.
- A 73% reduction of cardiac arrest rate per 1000 admissions from 6.27% to 1.71%.

Learning from practice

- It is important that staff have continuous training and reminders to complete PAR scores and to escalate care appropriately in line with NICE guidance.
- It is also noted that performance can only be maintained through continuous audit and attention.

Identifying a high-quality evidence base

CHAPTER 3

Paul Chrisp[1] and Sara Twaddle[2]

[1]Programme Director, Medicines and Prescribing Centre, National Institute for Health and Care Excellence, Manchester, UK

[2]Director, Scottish Intercollegiate Guidelines Network (SIGN), Healthcare Improvement Scotland, Edinburgh, UK

Introduction

As outlined in Chapter 1, the first step if you are aiming to improve the quality of health care is to identify the best available evidence-based guidance. As a health care professional, you will be bombarded on a daily basis with evidence from a variety of sources of varying quality. For busy practitioners, therefore, there is a need for a simple, efficient means of sifting this information to identify high-quality evidence to support the delivery of high-quality, effective and safe patient care.

With a specific focus on guidance, this chapter outlines some of the issues around the quality of evidence and its assessment: how and where to identify high-quality evidence; and what to consider when making evidence-based decisions. Case studies are used to highlight some of the key points.

Why it is important to seek high-quality evidence

The use of evidence in health care is well established. It sprang from the observation in the 1970s that there was wide variation in health care delivery: the realisation that there was a gap between what was practised and what was effective when assessed in controlled studies, and the lag between research results finding their way into practice. Against a backdrop of increasing costs of health care, it was clear that a more rational

Achieving High Quality Care: Practical Experience from NICE, First Edition.
Edited by Gillian Leng, Val Moore and Sasha Abraham.
© 2014 John Wiley & Sons, Ltd. Published 2014 by John Wiley & Sons, Ltd.

approach to health care was required. The response was for health care professionals to base their decisions on the best available evidence. This approach of evidence-based medicine, defined as *the conscientious, explicit, and judicious use of current best evidence in making decisions about the care of individual patients*, really took root in the early 1990s. Although the gap between evidence and practice as a result of the move to evidence-based health care has narrowed, the need to base practice on evidence has been made more acute by an acceleration in expenditure, fuelled by an increase in the cost of health care technologies and an increase in the number of older people and those living with long-term conditions.

How does guidance support evidence-based medicine?

Guidance can be defined as statements that include recommendations intended to optimise patient care that are informed by a systematic review of evidence and an assessment of the benefits and harms of alternative care options. Guidance is therefore seen as the most obvious place to enable evidence-based medicine to be implemented in practice.

Consequently, over the last 20 years, the number of guidelines has increased significantly. The US Agency for Healthcare Research and Quality's (AHRQ) National Guideline Clearinghouse contains nearly 2700 clinical practice guidelines, and the Guidelines International Network's (G-I-N) database lists more than 3700. This in itself poses problems for health care professionals as they struggle to know which guidance is relevant to them, and which are the most important among a large selection of guidelines and advice. The most useful information needs to be relevant, valid and easy to find (Figure 3.1) [1].

How can the standard of guidance development be checked?

It is recognised that clinical guidance can be of variable quality, both in methodology and in reporting, and a number of appraisal instruments

$$\text{Usefulness} = \frac{\text{Validity} \times \text{Relevance}}{\text{Effort}}$$

Fig. 3.1 What makes medical information practically useful. (Source: Shaughnessy *et al.* 1994 [1]. Reproduced with permission of Frontline Medical Communications.)

and standards have been developed to tackle the growing problem of multiple guidelines of variable quality. Although they differ in *how*, all look at 10 dimensions of *what* constitutes guideline quality:

- Validity
- Reliability/reproducibility
- Clinical applicability
- Clinical flexibility
- Clarity
- Scheduled review
- Development team
- Implementation
- Dissemination
- Evaluation.

A set of practical standards for guideline development has been proposed by the G-I-N that addresses these essential elements (Table 3.1) [2].

Clinicians can use the Appraisal of Guidelines Research and Evaluation (AGREE) instrument [3] to assess the quality of guidance development. The AGREE instrument evaluates all 10 of the key dimensions of guideline quality and has been internationally validated. It is an easy-to-use tool that covers 23 items across six domains to assess the quality of guideline development and the quality of reporting. Guidance developers can use the instrument to ensure their processes are robust, and health care professionals can use it to judge the quality of the processes used to develop guidance before putting it into practice. It also has utility for policy-makers and for educators to teach appraisal skills. The instrument was updated in 2010, widening its scope, making its purpose more explicit and modifying some wording of criteria [4].

It is estimated that an assessment of guidance using AGREE II will take on average 1.5 hours and should be conducted by at least two and ideally four assessors, which may limit its practical usefulness for busy clinicians.

How does guidance perform against these standards?

There has been limited and inconsistent improvement in the quality of guidance over the past two decades [5, 6]. In particular, the quality of processes to ensure editorial independence, appropriate stakeholder involvement and applicability has remained low, and only moderate advances have been made around rigour of development. Guidelines in oncology, internal medicine, musculoskeletal and paediatrics rate higher in the processes used to describe scope, rigour of development, clarity and independence. As rigour of development could be seen as the strongest indicator of quality, the fact that processes here tend only to be rated as moderate

Table 3.1 Standards for high-quality guidelines

Composition of guideline development group	A guideline development panel should include diverse and relevant stakeholders, such as health professionals, methodologists, topic experts and patients
Decision-making process	A guideline should describe the process used to reach consensus among the panel members and, if applicable, approval by the sponsoring organisation. This process should be established before the start of guideline development
Conflicts of interest	A guideline should include disclosure of the financial and nonfinancial conflicts of interest for members of the guideline development group. The guideline should also describe how any identified conflicts were recorded and resolved
Scope of guideline	A guideline should specify its objectives and scope
Methods	A guideline should clearly describe the methods used for the guideline development in detail
Evidence reviews	Guideline developers should use systematic evidence review methods to identify and evaluate evidence related to the guideline topic
Guideline recommendations	A guideline recommendation should be clearly stated and based on scientific evidence of benefits, harms and, if possible, costs
Rating of evidence and recommendations	A guideline should use a rating system to communicate the quality and reliability of both the evidence and the strength of its recommendations
Peer review and stakeholder consultation	Review by external stakeholders should be conducted before guideline publication
Guideline expiration and updating	A guideline should include an expiration date and/or describe the process that the guideline groups will use to update recommendations
Financial support and sponsoring organisation	A guideline should disclose financial support for the development of both the evidence review and the guideline recommendations

Source: Qaseem *et al.* 2012 [2]. Reproduced with permission of American College of Physicians.

over almost two decades is a particular concern. Guidance from governmental and international institutions has better processes than that from medical societies in all domains except, perhaps surprisingly, editorial independence.

So despite the availability of standards and appraisal tools, guidance quality is still often suboptimal. This may go some way to explain the observations that clinical guidelines have limited effects on outcomes. Other explanations include non-compliance with guidance recommendations as a result of being unable to find the most relevant, reliable guidance amid the clutter.

Can the ability of guidance to improve patient outcomes be checked?

Although the AGREE tool can be used to assess the quality of guidelines in terms of methodology and reporting, it does not assess the impact of implementation of the recommendations on patient outcomes. In this, AGREE is not alone – there is lack of a simple tool that assesses the usefulness of guidance recommendations.

It is nevertheless important to remember that patient outcomes are dependent on many variables other than the quality of care, and process standards have been suggested as the optimal way to manage health care performance. Quality standards that focus on the treatment and prevention of different diseases and conditions, supported by indicators and incentives to sustain improvements, can be used to link outcomes with high-quality evidence. NICE has developed a suite of quality standards based on high-quality guidance.

How can high-quality evidence be found?

Health care professionals frequently comment that the knowledge and information they need to deliver excellent care can be too hard to find. A web-based service, NICE Evidence (www.evidence.nhs.uk), was launched (as NHS Evidence) in May 2009 by NICE to help health care professionals quickly identify the most useful information they need [7]. Users of NICE Evidence can search for and quickly retrieve the most relevant information and recognise the most valid (i.e. trusted) guidance through an Accreditation Mark (Figure 3.2). The Accreditation Mark is awarded to organisations that meet a set of criteria, or standards, for guidance development.

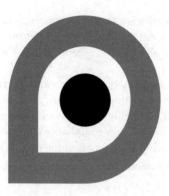

Fig. 3.2 The NICE Accreditation Mark.

What is NICE accreditation?

The NICE accreditation programme aims to raise the quality of information used by health care professionals by evaluating the processes used by organisations to produce guidance and recognise those that meet a set of criteria. The criteria are based on AGREE II, as this was the tool found to be the most suitable out of those reviewed, based on applicability of criteria, credibility and international recognition. NICE accreditation uses 25 criteria organised into six domains (Table 3.2). The minor adaptations made to the AGREE II criteria were to accommodate the wider range of guidance covered by NICE accreditation and to give a clearer focus on process rather than individual pieces of guidance. The accreditation criteria are used to assess the processes used by guidance developers, and compliance is rated as met, not fully met/uncertain, or not met. An independent Accreditation Advisory Committee reviews the information and makes an accreditation recommendation.

To be eligible to apply for NICE accreditation, an organisation must produce guidance that meets the definition of systematically developed statements to guide decisions about appropriate health and social care to improve individual and population health and well-being. In addition to clinical and other practice guidelines, this definition, therefore, encompasses the range of guidance and advice likely to be important to those providing or funding health care; this includes referral guidelines, public health guidelines, clinical summaries and best practice statements. Individual guidance products that are produced using an accredited process are eligible to display the Accreditation Mark, but NICE does not evaluate the content of each individual piece of guidance produced by an organisation. A summary of the steps in the accreditation process is

Table 3.2 NICE accreditation domains and criteria

Domain	Criteria
1. **Scope and purpose** is concerned with the overall aim of the guidance, the specific health questions and the target population	These criteria consider whether the guidance producer has a policy in place and adhered to that requires them to explicitly detail: 1.1 The overall objective of the guidance 1.2 The clinical, health care or social questions covered by the guidance 1.3 The population and/or target audience to whom the guidance applies 1.4 The producer ensures that the guidance includes clear recommendations in reference to specific clinical, health care or social circumstances
2. **Stakeholder involvement** focuses on the extent to which the guidance represents the views of its intended users and those affected by the guidance (patients and service users)	These criteria consider whether the guidance producer has a policy in place and adhered to that means it includes the following: 2.1 Individuals from all relevant stakeholder groups including patient groups in developing guidance 2.2 Patient and service user representatives seek patients' views and preferences in developing guidance 2.3 Representative intended users in developing guidance
3. **Rigour of development** relates to the process used to gather and synthesise information and the methods used to formulate recommendations and update them	These criteria consider whether the guidance producer has a clear policy in place and adhered to that means it includes the following: 3.1 Requires the guidance producer to use systematic methods to search for evidence and provide details of the search strategy 3.2 Requires the guidance producer to state the criteria and reasons for inclusion or exclusion of evidence identified by the evidence review 3.3 Describes the strengths and limitations of the body of evidence and acknowledges any areas of uncertainty 3.4 Describes the method used to arrive at recommendations (for example, a voting system or formal consensus techniques like Delphi consensus) 3.5 Requires the guidance producers to consider the health benefits, side effects and risks in formulating recommendations

(continued overleaf)

Table 3.2 (*continued*)

Domain	Criteria
	3.6 Describes the processes of external peer review 3.7 Describes the process of updating guidance and maintaining and improving guidance quality
4. **Clarity and presentation** deal with the language and format of the guidance	These criteria consider whether the guidance producer ensures the following: 4.1 The recommendations are specific, unambiguous and clearly identifiable 4.2 The different options for management of the condition or options for intervention are clearly presented 4.3 The date of search, the date of publication or last update and the proposed date for review are clearly stated 4.4 The content and style of the guidance are suitable for the specified target audience. If the public, patients or service users are part of this audience, the language should be appropriate
5. **Applicability** deals with the likely organisational, behavioural and cost implications of applying the guidance	These criteria consider whether the guidance producer routinely considers the following: 5.1 Publishing support tools to aid implementation of guidance 5.2 Discussion of potential organisational and financial barriers in applying its recommendations 5.3 Review criteria for monitoring and/or audit purposes within each product
6. **Editorial independence** is concerned with the independence of the recommendations, acknowledgement of possible conflicts of interest, the credibility of the guidance in general and their recommendations in particular	These criteria consider whether the guidance producer considers the following parameters: 6.1 Ensures editorial independence from the funding body 6.2 Is transparent about the funding mechanisms for its guidance 6.3 Records and states any potential conflicts of interest of individuals involved in developing the recommendations 6.4 Takes account of any potential for bias in the conclusions or recommendations of the guidance

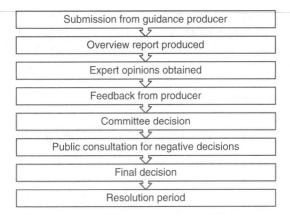

Fig. 3.3 Outline of the NICE accreditation process.

shown in Figure 3.3. As at the end of December 2012, 60 processes had been evaluated in the programme and over 4000 pieces of guidance on NICE Evidence display the Accreditation Mark.

So rather than having to conduct their own assessment of a guideline using AGREE II, the Accreditation Mark offers busy clinicians a quick and easy way of identifying a comprehensive range of guidance that has been produced using a high-quality process. Case study 3.1 illustrates the breadth of guidance covered by accreditation from national guidance developers producing a large number of guidelines across a broad range of conditions to smaller, more specialist organisations that produce guidance for very specific conditions or settings. As we have seen, the proliferation of the internet and its increased use in the clinical situation potentially offer quick and simple access to evidence for health care professionals. There is a need, however, to filter this information to identify high-quality material. Case study 3.2 gives an example and some of the practical issues encountered.

What does NICE accreditation say about guidance quality?

Results from the NICE accreditation programme indicate that the criteria least likely to be met (judged as those that were not fully met or not met in 15% or more of cases) are consideration of patient views, processes for inclusion and exclusion of evidence, methods to make recommendations, process for updating guidance, date of search, publication or last update, and review date and discussion of potential barriers to implementation.

Deficiencies in detailing the clinical questions of guidance, describing the patient group/target audience, methods to describe the strengths and limitations in the evidence and accounting for bias are more likely to be found in processes that are not accredited, indicating strong predictors of poor-quality guidance. These results are consistent with the observations of guideline quality discussed earlier.

What if there is no relevant high-quality guidance?

It might be the case that a search of NICE Evidence fails to identify accredited guidance that is relevant to a particular clinical question or local setting, or in fact relevant guidance that could be appraised using AGREE II has not actually been published. In these circumstances, clinicians may need to develop guidance specific to their question or setting. The G-I-N or AGREE II standards should be used as a basis for the development process.

How to get high-quality evidence into practice?

Figure 3.4 summarises the steps in identifying a high-quality evidence base to improve the quality of care. Finding relevant, trustworthy guidance is just one aspect of getting evidence into practice. Looking back to the definition of evidence-based medicine from earlier in this chapter, the other aspect is that of evidence-based individual decision-making. This recognises that, unlike guidance which is by its very nature indirect, health care professionals directly responsible for patient care need to implement and apply evidence-based decisions to individual patients. Chapter 4 discusses the key challenges to implementation and effective interventions.

Learning from practice

1 The volume of guidance is increasing and its quality is variable.
2 A range of tools and standards, such as AGREE II, is available to help practitioners check guidance quality, just as standards can be used to critically appraise studies.
3 These tools address a common set of features of guidance development, are straightforward to use, and can be used to develop local guidelines if no relevant high-quality guidance exists.
4 NICE accreditation also offers a quick way to identify trusted guidance, which is the first step in improving the quality of care.

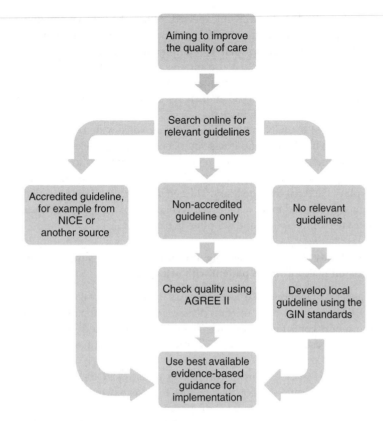

Fig. 3.4 Summary of steps to identify a high-quality evidence base to improve the quality of care.

Case Study 3.1: Different guidance producers evaluated using NICE accreditation

An established guidance producer covering a wide span of topics, the Scottish Intercollegiate Guidelines Network (SIGN), was set up by the Medical Royal Colleges and Faculties in Scotland in 1993 to produce evidence-based multidisciplinary guidelines for NHS Scotland. Already well known and attracting around 20 million hits on its website (www.sign.ac.uk) every year, there was initial reluctance to put SIGN forward for accreditation by NICE Evidence because of concerns about the burden of the process itself and uncertainty about the benefits to such an established organisation. Nevertheless, SIGN decided to proceed and found that the process itself was considerably less burdensome than feared and the benefits were unexpected. Although SIGN's methodology is designed around the AGREE criteria, the accreditation analysis revealed some processes that would benefit from being strengthened or applied more rigorously, prompting a review of processes. SIGN now displays the NICE Accreditation Mark on its website and on its guidelines and has observed an increase in the number of visitors to its website routed via NICE Evidence.

In contrast to SIGN that produces guidance on a wide range of topics, the Children's Brain Tumour Research Centre only produces the Diagnosis of Brain Tumours in Children guideline. The process to develop the guideline was accredited in 2011 and the website of the research centre displays the Accreditation Mark. The benefits of accreditation are again a higher profile and more widespread recognition of a good-quality guideline, facilitating uptake and adoption in practice.

Case Study 3.2: A GP looking for information to support clinical decision-making with a patient with osteopaenia

A general practitioner (GP) receives a dual-energy X-ray absorptiometry (DEXA) report on bone mineral density for a postmenopausal woman. The report confirms osteopenia. The GP is keen to find good quality, evidence-based information on appropriate treatment and scanning intervals.

A simple Google search of *osteopenia management* identifies 869 000 pages of information. Narrowing this to a search on *osteopenia management guidelines* throws up 2040 pages of information, ranging from guidelines to primary research papers, pharmaceutical industry material and personal stories. In a clinical setting this is clearly not a useful approach and the GP is left wondering which colleagues from medical school to call on for advice.

Collections of guidelines

The GP can search databases of clinical guidelines, and then use AGREE II to conduct his/her own assessment of clinical guidelines identified in this way.

Using the example of management of osteopaenia management, a search of the AHRQ database in February 2013 found 36 entries. The GP is now getting fed up!

NICE Evidence and accreditation

Accredited guidelines appear at the top of search results on NICE Evidence, saving time in identifying the most trusted sources of guidance.

Identifying and using guidelines that carry a *kitemark* such as the NICE Accreditation Mark can go a long way to help busy professionals overcome both barriers of poor quality and too much information.

Using the example of management of osteopaenia, a search of NICE Evidence in February 2013 found 486 entries. Using the filter, the GP was able to identify relevant guidelines with an Accreditation Mark. The GP downloads the relevant information and plans care for the patient.

What if there is more than one good-quality source?

In the earlier example, the GP was able to identify a single good-quality guideline that addressed their information needs. However, as more guidance becomes available and standards rise, the probability of different recommendations based on the same, or very similar, good-quality evidence becomes a possibility.

This issue arises because the development of evidence-based advice is not simply a systematic review of existing evidence from which a recommendation emerges. Instead, guidance development requires evidence to be interpreted in the light of local circumstances, patient preferences, epidemiology, resource constraints and health systems. In the United Kingdom, setting recommendations from NICE and SIGN on the same topic may differ to some degree, reflecting the divergence of the two health care systems.

This may pose a problem if there are differences in recommendations from accredited sources. In such circumstances, our GP may wish to consider the following questions to guide them to the most relevant recommendations:

- Is the guidance relevant for my health care setting?
- Which is most relevant to this specific patient, taking into account their condition, values and preferences?
- Which is the most recent guidance?
- Are the recommendations implementable in my practice?
- Who was involved in developing the guidance?

What if there is a relevant guideline but it is out of date?

An additional issue that may arise is that of timeliness. Good practice, as identified by the standards for guidance development, is that there is a clear procedure for updating it and for maintaining and improving its quality. In practice, most guidance developers will assess the need for review on a regular basis (usually at least every 3 years), and a review would also take place if the evidence base has changed sufficiently to alter the recommendations. Thus, apparently *old* guidance may contain valid recommendations. If our GP came across such a situation, they should therefore check the review dates and plans for update to check if it has been reviewed recently and is current. If not, he or she may be using outdated practices to manage the patient, and they should check other sources for important new evidence that may affect guidance recommendations.

References

1 Shaughnessy, A.F., Slawson, D.C. & Bennett, J.H. (1994) Becoming an information master: a guidebook to the medical information jungle. *Journal of Family Practice*, **39**, 489–499.
2 Qaseem, A., Forland, F., Macbeth, F. *et al.* (2012) Guidelines International Network: toward international standards for clinical practice guidelines. *Annals of Internal Medicine*, **156**, 525–531.
3 AGREE Collaboration (2003) Development and validation of an international appraisal instrument for assessing the quality of clinical practice guidelines: the AGREE project. *Quality & Safety in Health Care*, **12**, 18–23.
4 Brouwers, M.C., Kho, M.E., Browman, G.P. *et al.* (2010) AGREE II: advancing guideline development, reporting and evaluation in health care. *CMAJ*, **182**, E839–E842.
5 Alonso-Coello, P., Irfan, A., Solá, I. *et al.* (2010) The quality of clinical practice guidelines over the last two decades: a systematic review of guideline appraisal studies. *Quality & Safety in Health Care*, **19**, 1–7.
6 Kung J, Miller RR, Mackowiak PA. Failure of clinical practice guidelines to meet Institute of Medicine standards: two more decades of little, if any, progress. *Archives of Internal Medicine* 2012;**172**:1628–163310.1001/2013.jamainternmed.56.
7 Leng, G.C. (2009) NHS Evidence: better and faster access to information. *Lancet*, **373**, 1502–1504.

Further reading

Eddy DM. Practice policies: where do they come from? *JAMA: The Journal of the American Medical Association* 1990;**263**; 1265, 1269, 1275.
Eddy, D.M. (2005) Evidence-based medicine: a unified approach. *Health Affairs*, **24**, 9–17.
Institute of Medicine (2011) *Clinical Practice Guidelines We Can Trust*. National Academies Press, Washington, DC.
Sackett DL Rosenberg, W.M.C., Gray, J.A., *et al.* Evidence-based medicine: what it is and what it isn't. *BMJ: British Medical Journal* 1996;**312**:71-72.
Vlayen, J., Aertgeerts, B., Hannes, K. *et al.* (2005) A systematic review of appraisal tools for clinical practice guidelines: multiple similarities and one common deficit. *International Journal for Quality in Health Care*, **17**, 235–242.
Wennberg, J.E. & Gittlesohn, A. (1973) Small area variations in health care delivery. *Science*, **82**, 1102–1108.

Example in Practice

Finding a way through guidance on pre-hospital care across South West England

The acquisition of a local ambulance service by an existing ambulance service NHS Foundation Trust in the South West in February 2013 provided an opportunity to harmonise and advance clinical practice. NICE guidelines were central to the process.

The new service successfully brought together clinical expertise from the two organisations with a focus on delivering evidence-based care from day 1, resulting in consistent and enhanced care for patients across the South West.

> Changing the clinical practice of so many clinicians across a large area is challenging: effective communication is vital.
>
> Source: Adrian South, Deputy Clinical Director.

Finding a way through guidance

The ambition was to harmonise clinical practice from day 1 – a challenge with 3000 staff working across 120 sites. Both services had previously used a system of clinical notices to disseminate NICE guidelines to staff. It was difficult to keep up with over 30 annual updates and memorise the detail of many of the guidelines. Over 450 clinical documents had been published by both organisations in the last 6 years. The information was also difficult to remember; for example, the safe application of the paediatric fever traffic light system required clinicians to memorise 46 criteria.

Applying guidelines in a fast-moving, unpredictable pre-hospital environment presents unique challenges for ambulance services in the United Kingdom. A radically new approach was needed to ensure that ambulance clinicians on the front line had quick access to key clinical information. A standard, concise and easy to access resource written by ambulance clinicians, for ambulance clinicians, has resulted in a range of benefits, including better availability of guidance out in the field, a higher profile of evidence-based practice, improvements in the implementation of guidance and, most importantly, improved care.

Smart access on the move

In December 2012, every ambulance clinician was issued with a clinical guidelines folder, developed by the senior clinical teams working together to review guidance. Baseline assessment identified 24 areas where further guidance was required. Six senior paramedics combined the best clinical practice from both organisations with the latest evidence base. The guidelines had to be accessible, concise and provide practical support to ambulance clinicians of all grades. During January 2013, staff reviewed the guidelines to ensure that they could be fully implemented from day 1.

The guidelines were published on the services intranet and websites, with staff encouraged to download the documents onto their smartphones. Where available on ambulances, existing rugged laptops were used to further enhance access, with officers also using an iPad App. A key challenge for staff working remotely across sites was to be able to rapidly access advice and clarification. The implementation was supported by the senior clinical team, spending a week in the field providing information sessions at 11 main ambulance stations. An on-call advice email service provided access to a member of the senior clinical team to answer questions within an hour, 08:00–23:00, 7 days a week.

Monitoring improvement in outcomes

The successful implementation of the guidelines will be monitored using a combination of clinical audit, incident report review and analysis of serious incidents. An analysis of the serious incidents reviewed over the past year demonstrated that the new clinical guidelines had been available and applied at the time of the incident, all applicable cases would have been averted. It is hoped that the project will further improve patient safety, and further decrease the number of serious incidents.

A wide range of relevant NICE guidance is now firmly embedded across the organisation, with an accompanying increase in the profile of NICE resources.

Learning from practice

- It is important to demonstrate the advantage of aiming for harmonised clinical care from day 1, when previous ambulance mergers have used the approach of harmonising care over the first 1–2 years.
- The use of multiple implementation methods has also contributed to the success of the project, which took just 6 months from start to completion.
- Although this example is focused on pre-hospital services, this learning may be relevant to other organisations or services that are anticipating merger or reconfiguration.

Key challenges to implementation and effective interventions

CHAPTER 4

Elaine Whitby[1] and Julie Royce[2]

[1]Education & Support, National Institute for Health and Care Excellence, Manchester, UK
[2]Implementation Support, National Institute for Health and Care Excellence, London, UK

Introduction

Combined with judgement and knowledge of the local context, who would argue with the principle that we should base our decisions on the best available evidence of what works? Implementing evidence-based guidance is essential for good quality care. Just as NICE guidance is evidence based, there are also established and emerging evidence-based frameworks and approaches to implementation that can help to inform practical actions.

The best guidance is only beneficial to patients once implemented; however, introducing guidance into clinical practice requires knowledge, skill, collaboration and a systematic approach. Responsibility for implementation of guidance and identification of the barriers resides with the implementation lead and team.

When any implementation project is introduced, it is likely to have an impact on numerous people, processes and systems. Some of these will be planned, and some will be unplanned and emerge as implementation progresses. The relationship between your project and others will be dynamic. This chapter seeks to explore some of the interconnections across systems, highlight types of barriers or facilitators to implementation you may encounter, and outline a systematic approach to designing interventions to address barriers.

Firstly, let us make clear what we mean by implementation. We mean an active, planned process (or multiple processes) designed to get best

Achieving High Quality Care: Practical Experience from NICE, First Edition.
Edited by Gillian Leng, Val Moore and Sasha Abraham.
© 2014 John Wiley & Sons, Ltd. Published 2014 by John Wiley & Sons, Ltd.

practice, based on guidance, routinely embedded in day-to-day activity. This spans the period from first encountering and considering guidance to it being fully embedded into the norms and rituals of everyday policy and practice.

In reality, there may be multiple levels of implementation activity, such as policy or structural work ongoing at national, regional and health economy levels. In addition, provider organisations may have designated quality leads that provide the infrastructure to support new guidance, and individually practitioners and teams may also have their own processes for incorporating guidance into front line practice. This chapter will prompt you to consider the levels of individual, group or team, organisation and the larger system and how they may interact with and influence your implementation work [1].

Understanding the different levels supported by a systematic approach to implementation is advised. Put simply, this involves assessing, planning, engaging, executing, reflecting and evaluating (Figure 4.1). In reality, these rarely occur in a linear fashion and often involve cyclical or incremental approaches. In Chapter 6, further reflection is given on this kind of quality improvement, or audit, cycle. Be under no illusion, implementation is challenging; it is common to move back and forth between assessment, planning and implementation. Setbacks and surprises may be encountered – it is important not to be put off, but to be prepared.

Not all of the elements outlined in this chapter will apply to all implementation projects – barriers in one project may differ greatly from those in another. Also, if the changes required affect only a single clinical team, this will require different considerations and resources than if implementation requires change across multiple professional and organisational boundaries. There are no magic bullets. Each implementation project will differ and will require customised interventions for success, so understanding your starting point and planning accordingly cannot be underestimated.

What are the main factors that will influence an implementation project?

What are the context and resource issues to consider?

Understanding the wider context within which an implementation project is introduced is essential. Facilitators or barriers to success can include motivation and goals, availability of resources, decision-making processes and structural or policy initiatives such as financial incentives and disincentives. For example, at the wider system level, heath care

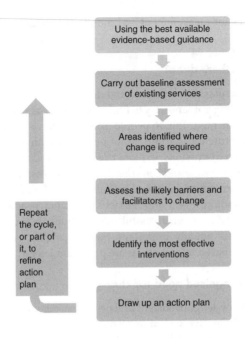

Fig. 4.1 Key stages in the implementation process.

systems undergoing significant organisational change may by necessity have to focus on establishing structure or governance processes. Changes to clinical pathways, while important, may not be the main priority, or the decision-making arrangements to *sign off* the project may be in a state of flux. Conversely a team who have experienced a very positive improvement in their outcomes for patients may be buoyed by their success and eager to develop further. Be aware of and seek opportunities. If the project is a good fit with organisational developments and wider policy agendas, it may have more chance of success. If it does not, be aware and look for opportunities where things do fit and make these into an opportunity. Swimming with the tide of team, organisational and national objectives are often easier than swimming against.

At a practical level, understanding available resources is also required. This may include staffing skills and capacity as well as equipment and ongoing costs to support implementation and delivery of the guidance. Resources to support implementation should also be considered. If this is a significant change programme, it is likely to require board or very senior manager level support and endorsement, investment in clinical leadership and project management, facilitated time for staff to meet and resources for measurement and monitoring progress as outlined in Chapter 2.

What have others done?

Be aware of similar developments and do not reinvent the wheel. If you are implementing guidance, try to find other organisations that may have already implemented. Talk to people from outside your team or organisation and capture ideas, examples of protocols, pathways or other best practice. In the discussions, explore *what* people did and also *how* they approached the change and consider these in your own plans. Acquiring protocols, education tools and so on can be very helpful but exploring and understanding levers and barriers that other people encountered and the successful or unsuccessful interventions they used to achieve their change are equally important. Some examples of local learning from evidence-based interventions are presented later in this chapter.

Is there a recognised need for change?

Generating knowledge of current practice is a precursor to changing practice. Ideally those involved in or affected by the change should have a shared understanding of the current situation and agree that there is a need for change and develop the necessary changes. For example, if doctors, nurses, managers and administrative staff on a ward all believe that recommendations from guidance will make a positive difference to their practice and to patient care, successful implementation is more likely. Most people strive to provide a good service and believe they are doing so. They may not see a need for change, or the change proposed may seem so disruptive to the current ways of working that the work required appears to outweigh the benefits. If so, engaging them successfully in implementation is far less likely.

Consider using readily available data to assess the service, for example, benchmarked performance data may indicate areas for improvement that can be further explored. Guidance can then be used to inform the improvements. A range of other methods for assessing current practice are available such as a review of incidents or critical case review of patients whose trajectory of care has not gone smoothly. Clinical audit is another option. NICE produces baseline assessment or gap analysis tools for clinical guidance that may save time for those working locally in the NHS.

How to engage and influence?

Working together helps build trust and understanding and generates shared knowledge. The process of achieving this should not be underestimated. If involving people in the change process is so important, then how can this be done? Identifying and engaging stakeholders, developing shared understanding and fostering commitment across disciplines requires flexibility and adapting to the context.

Effective communication and influence will be required for implementation. It is acknowledged that social and professional networks exert powerful influence on the adoption (or non-adoption) of innovations by individuals. Different groups have different types of networks, for instance, doctors tend to operate in informal networks with other doctors and are heavily influenced through colleagues. Informal networks often comprise individuals of similar professional backgrounds. This may mean that nurses, allied health professionals, doctors, managers and other specialists, for example audit or information experts, may all be influenced primarily by their own disciplines and professional colleagues and this can limit implementation [2, 3].

In addition, health care disciplines are often educated separately, drawing on differing published sources of evidence; and opportunities to participate in multiprofessional fora are limited. Where they do exist, for instance through clinical networks, they may be dominated by one professional group.

Promoting discussion of how to improve practice and services in multi professional fora as part of an implementation process can, therefore, be a useful mechanism to promote change. This enables knowledge transfer across the professional disciplines and enables all elements of the pathway of care to be considered. Creating specific project groups, utilising existing meetings and *ad hoc* opportunities can all contribute.

Some roles are considered useful in assisting the transfer of information across professional boundaries. Commonly called *boundary spanners* or *knowledge brokers*, people in these roles often work between networks and support relationships and facilitate knowledge transfer across social and professional boundaries. The role is both complex and contextual, with some individuals adopting whatever roles and approaches are needed to bring about the necessary change [4]. Such knowledge brokers may be formal roles identified by, for example, a title such as coordinator or project lead often seen in clinical or research networks [5]. Identification of colleagues who link with both your team and other groups or organisations is worthwhile as they may be influential in the change process.

The use of champions or opinion leaders is another strategy often used to promote implementation of good practice, although of course opinion leaders can hold views contrary to the evidence. These may either be national leaders or locally nominated champions for different developments or groups. While winning hearts and minds is crucial, the role of champions and opinion leaders is not as straightforward as it may seem. *Expert* opinion leaders are those with authority and status who are able to explain and respond to challenge effectively such as the appointed clinical champions mentioned earlier. However, peer opinion leaders can also be influential. These are viewed by their colleagues as someone to whom they can relate and who is perceived to have a close understanding of the work under consideration [6, 7]. Individuals are more likely to adopt an innovation if people with whom they have good, trustworthy interpersonal relationships support the innovation. If support for guidance is not provided or opinion leaders are indifferent, this may limit uptake.

The views of the main professional bodies should also be considered, for instance, are they consistent with the implementation programme? National or local policies may act as levers and individual disciplines may be more influenced by literature from their respective professional bodies, again demonstrating the need for a range of positive opinion leaders and knowledge brokers.

How to move forward?

A review of theories related to behaviour change proposes an over arching model (Figure 4.2) showing that behaviour occurs as an interaction

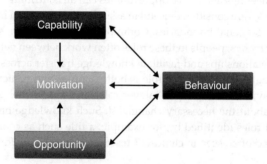

Fig. 4.2 The relationship between motivation and behaviour change. (Source: Michie 2011 [8]. Reproduced with permission of Professor Susan Michie.)

between capability, motivation and opportunity, and that if capability and opportunity are increased, this will impact on motivation [8].

In practical terms, improving individual capability may be achieved through developing knowledge and/or skills, and confidence in a particular activity increases motivation to work at increasing capabilities. Opportunity refers to the wider environment, such as availability of local project management support or identifying and joining a wider network-based programme working with peers and enabling information and resource sharing and potentially wider influence.

This behaviour change model is premised on the concept that improving the implementation of guidance depends on behaviour change, and that to do this successfully, it is necessary to consider the following conditions:

- understand current practice and identify the reasons for not implementing change;
- describe the behaviours that need to be changed, being specific about who needs to change what behaviour and in what circumstances;
- select appropriate interventions to address the specific behaviour changes required.

The sections that follow elaborate on these important stages.

How to assess current barriers and facilitators?

Effective assessment is essential to understand the various system elements and plan the interventions that will support guidance implementation. The assessment should include barriers and facilitators, followed by a plan of interventions tailored to the identified barriers as this is more likely to improve professional practice than no intervention or by simply disseminating guidelines. There is no evidence to help determine the best way to tailor any interventions, but it is reasonable to employ low-cost-tailored interventions to increase the likelihood of success [9].

It is also important to note, however, that no interventions are effective under all circumstances, and the effect of any one intervention is modest. Skilled analysis of each implementation programme to ensure good assessment and interventions targeted at specific barriers and appropriate to the professional groups and context can aid successful implementation.

How to find out more about behaviours and barriers?

There are many methods for identifying potential barriers, and depending on programme size and resources some may be more feasible than others. These might include individual interviews or conversations, focus groups or building structured time into team, network or project group meetings, surveys or direct observations. The facilitator of any implementation project will need to use their judgement about how best to identify the behaviours and barriers, given their understanding of the context and available resources. Some tools are available to help teams to appraise their current situation.

Once identified, it may be helpful to map barriers at multiple levels of the health care system as outlined in the example as shown in Box 4.1.

Box 4.1 Example of possible barriers to change mapped at multiple levels

Individual

Belief that current practice is of high quality, therefore no reason to change.
Lack of skills or confidence in new techniques.

Team

Variation in practice between members of the team: each have their personal preferences.
A single individual or discipline dominates the development agenda.

Organisation

Re-organisation resulting in changing staff and structures at senior management level, and unclear who has authority to endorse the changes.
Lack of resources for establishing new clinics.

Wider context

Inconsistencies between national guidance developed by different organisations.
Financial disincentives.

How to prioritise action?

A useful next step may be to decide which barriers can most readily be addressed. For instance, regarding a re-organisation (see Box 4.1), you may have to wait until the staff structure is in place to identify the responsible senior manager. Regarding conflicting guidance, while you are not able to change the guidance you may be able to get the team to compare and contrast strengths and applicability of both and to develop a local protocol.

Once you have identified the barriers that can be addressed, you need to identify which are highest priorities, focusing on those that need to be addressed before guidance implementation can progress.

What interventions should be used in the implementation plan?

Each implementation project will differ and will require bespoke interventions for success, and should be tailored towards the prospectively identified barriers and take account of available resources (Chapter 5 contains more information on making a business case for action). Having identified your priorities, Box 4.2 below outlines a range of possible interventions. Choose those that best address the identified barriers and may help to facilitate the required behaviour change. For many of these interventions, specific support tools are provided by NICE to facilitate change. These are available via the NICE website.

Remember that research shows that individual interventions alone may have small effects, and that combining methods may achieve a bigger overall impact on change.

Box 4.2 Interventions to help overcome barriers to change

Clinical audit

Clinical audit aims to improve patient care and outcomes through systematic review of care against explicit criteria, such as guidance recommendations. It includes the implementation of necessary changes and further clinical audit to confirm quality improvement.

What the research shows

Clinical audit and feedback can be effective in improving practice. Research shows that 'audit and feedback generally leads to small but potentially important improvements in professional practice. The effectiveness of audit and feedback seems to depend on baseline performance and how the feedback is provided'.

Examples from practice demonstrate that data alone may be insufficient to influence change, but belief in the audit processes used, clinician buy-in and credibility of the project lead will also have an impact [10].

Example from practice

A hospital in England uses clinical audit to support continuous improvement in its performance avoiding inadvertent hypothermia. The publication of a new NICE guideline on perioperative hypothermia acted as a catalyst for further improvement, stimulating a re-audit using the NICE clinical audit tool to check alignment with the NICE recommendations.

Challenges identified from the re-audit included coordinating the warming of patients along their whole journey and providing sufficient warming devices to implement this. The audit found that the responsibility of managing the warming of patients from wards to theatre pre-operatively and from recovery to ward was not clearly defined. Also, the cost of purchasing sufficient warming devices or equipment to maintain near normothermia outside theatres was found to be a perceived barrier. Coordination and education of staff in multiple areas in the hospital were also required.

Following this audit, the hospital's future development will focus on the phases of temperature control outside theatre and tackling the difficulties faced here. Potential additional investment may be made to enable this with increased warmers in recovery and more blankets for transfer to and from wards.

Education

Educational interventions can be used to address behaviour change including addressing such barriers as a lack of awareness, scepticism or misunderstanding, or a lack of knowledge or competency. They may take many forms, including the use of educational materials such as leaflets, podcasts, videos and online learning aids; events and meetings dedicated to meeting educational objectives; and outreach using trained individuals to visit health care professionals in their practice.

What the research shows

'When compared to no intervention, printed educational materials when used alone may have a beneficial effect on process outcomes but not on patient outcomes' [11].

'Educational outreach visits alone or when combined with other interventions have effects on prescribing that are relatively consistent and small, but potentially important. Their effects on other types of professional performance vary from small to modest improvements' [12].

'Educational meetings alone or combined with other interventions, can improve professional practice and health care outcomes for the patients. The effect is most likely to be small. Strategies to increase attendance at educational meetings, using mixed interactive and didactic formats, and focusing on outcomes that are likely to be perceived as serious may increase the effectiveness of educational meetings. Educational meetings alone are not likely to be effective for changing complex behaviours' [13].

Example from practice

A trust in the East of England aimed to improve the quality of decisions made between clinicians in 16 general practices and their patients with lower urinary tract symptoms. They identified that evidence-based pathways and GP education were not enough to change clinical behaviour across the board. A detailed evaluation of each clinician's referrals informed an initial audit that identified GP educational needs. This was used to inform feedback to individual clinicians. A series of educational events were delivered, supported by educational materials and patient decision aids, clinicians bimonthly feedback on their referrals and a local communications campaign.

Three-month audits revealed a 39% improvement in appropriate referrals. One year later, a re-audit showed an overall reduction in referrals resulting in over £28 000 annual saving.

Opinion leaders

Opinion leaders have influence to motivate and inspire health care professionals to achieve the best possible care for patients. They are well respected among their peers and act as role models for junior colleagues.

What the research shows

Research has identified that opinion leaders, either alone or in combination with other interventions, may assist implementation of evidence-based practice. However, unfortunately because of the nature of the studies, it is not possible to identify the most effective ways that opinion leaders can support implementation. The role of opinion leaders is complex; but the evidence supports that identification and use of credible, likeable and trustworthy opinion leaders to promote guidance implementation should be considered [7].

Example from practice

A critical care network working across two counties in England aimed to achieve 100% compliance with the NICE guidance on delirium. There was a lack of clinician interest in the condition as its relationship with organ failure was not understood, and there was scepticism regarding the evidence.

To address these barriers, the network carried out an audit using the NICE clinical audit tool. These results were analysed collaboratively and local action plans were devised. Action included an educational conference that was recognised for continuing professional development and the inclusion of a scoring box in the nursing team handover sheets.

This initiative was supported by an identified clinical champion who encouraged daily assessment on unit rounds.

The result of these interventions was increased recognition of delirium in organ failure by clinicians and the implementation of improvements in daily assessments and care planning.

Reminders

Reminders are designed to prompt a health professional to recall information and remind them to perform or avoid some action to aid individual patient care. They may take many forms – examples include posters, desk reminders and computer prompts.

What the research shows

Reminders can be moderately effective in changing behaviour, particularly when computer decision support is used to influence prescribing and the delivery of preventative care services. They are more effective if designed to specifically address barriers to change. There are concerns that computer decision support may not cope with the complexities of patient–doctor decision-making [14].

Example from practice

A large general practice in England aimed to improve the assessment of all febrile children, using all four assessment criteria recommended in NICE guidance as the baseline assessment showed that this was not happening.

To identify the reasons for this and barriers to change, a number of methods were used including a staff questionnaire, direct observation and leadership *walk arounds*. Barriers included a lack of equipment, a lack of awareness and concern about increasing the length of consultations.

This led to implementing a multi-faceted intervention which included: making the equipment available and putting the traffic light table on the practice intranet for ease of reference; a number of reminder interventions that included a visible prompt on the tympanic thermometer just below the screen with a picture of the child and a checklist; computer mouse mats with a picture of the same child having her temperature checked; a table of the normal values placed in each room; an electronic data recording algorithm with coding that prompted a *forcing* function to avoid omissions and, finally, a personalised postcard reminder for those persistently not conducting all four features of the assessment.

Data collected showed that improvements were made in conducting all four assessments, and it did not increase the length of consultation. More information on this example including additional interventions used is provided at the end of this chapter.

Patient-mediated strategies

Patient-mediated strategies focus on helping patients to influence good practice. For example, this could be by giving information to patients and the wider public, or through mass media advertising.

What the research shows

Passing information to patients through mass media may be effective in changing clinician behaviour, although it is unclear whether this effect is due to patients or clinicians themselves making use of the information; the methodological quality of studies in this area is low.

There is some evidence that providing educational materials for patients can help the implementation of guidelines. Direct-to-patient advertising by pharmaceutical companies appears to affect patient demand for drugs, but there are no rigorous evaluations of this. The impact of public reporting of clinician performance is unclear, although there is some evidence implying that it affects an organisation's behaviour [14].

Example from practice

A project in the North West of England aimed to improve engagement with respiratory patients to ensure that the agreed Chronic Obstructive Pulmonary

Disease (COPD) treatment standards were met when they visited any respiratory service in the North West. A core intervention for achieving this was the setting up of a patient leader programme.

Patient leaders were recruited from existing COPD patient groups and were given training to act as a representative for their locality or community working in collaboration with key agencies. Their role was to voice patient need, identify best practice examples and work in partnership with services to improve patient experience and outcomes. A link with their local service funder, responsible for contracting service provision in their area, was facilitated and supported – for example to participate in the training.

Audit of adherence suggests that improvements have been made and the patient leaders have responded positively to the initiative, perceiving that the impact has been greater than previous initiatives.

How to design the implementation project and evaluation?

Developing an implementation plan is the next step in the process. Robust planning including clarity of actions and responsibilities: *what, when, where, how* and *who* will aid implementation. Planning also needs to be realistic, taking into account resources and ensuring interventions are practical and appropriate for the degree of change required. Building in evaluation from the outset is also recommended.

Our experience and the literature tell us that it may be helpful to consider the following points to develop the implementation plan:

- Multiple interventions are likely to have greater impact than single interventions.
- Barriers and required behaviour change are likely to have been identified at multiple levels. Interventions should therefore be targeted at multiple levels. This could include policy change at organisational level, educational team meetings and individual skill-based activities.
- Involve the target groups in developing and implementing the plan. Multiprofessional meetings are useful to exchange and generate shared understanding, and collaboration should help to engender trust and stimulate cooperation. It will also enable the practical knowledge of the stakeholders to be taken into account to ensure the design of any new systems or processes are usable, practical and meet their needs.
- Where possible, build on existing activities. If there are already group meetings, consider how these can be utilised for project meetings or educational sessions.

- Consider measurable goals and how these will be monitored and evaluated. Where possible use existing data or measurement rather than add to the burden of data collection.
- If the project is of significant size, break it down into phases with clear goals so that milestones can be reached and acknowledged. This may build motivation and maintain momentum.

Summary overview

A systematic evidence-informed approach to implementation should be used to generate a change in practice. Each implementation project will differ and will require specific interventions for success. Consideration should be given to the multiple layers of the health care system including individual, team, organisational and wider levels. Evidence-based interventions include education, clinical audit, opinion leaders, reminders and patient-mediated approaches. Continuous assessment and review including ongoing engagement with stakeholders and the monitoring of progress will be essential – more on this last point will be found in Chapter 6.

Learning from practice

1 Multiple levels of the system and their interdependencies should be considered including individual, team, organisational and wider system levels.
2 A systematic approach to guidance implementation including the identification of barriers and facilitators should be adopted.
3 An explicit implementation programme using a range of evidence-based interventions to address the barriers will support effective implementation.
4 Implementation is unpredictable and requires ongoing assessment and flexibility to respond to changing circumstances.

References

1 Ferlie, E.B. and Shortell, S.M. (2001) Improving the quality of health care in the United Kingdom and the United States: a framework for change. *The Milbank Quarterly*, **79** (2), 281–315.
2 Greenhalgh, T., Robert, G., MacFarlane, F. *et al.* (2004) Diffusion of innovations in service organisations: systematic review and recommendations. *The Milbank Quarterly*, **82** (4), 581–629.

3 Ferlie, E., Fitzgerald, L., Wood, M. and Hawkins, C. (2005) The nonspread of innovations: the mediating role of professionals. *Academy of Management Journal*, **48** (1), 117–134.

4 Conklin, J., Lusk, E., Harris, M. and Stolle, P. (2013) Knowledge brokers in a knowledge network: the case of Seniors Health Research Transfer Network knowledge brokers. *Implementation Science*, **8**, 7.

5 Ferlie, E., Fitzgerald, L., McGivern, G. *et al.* (2013) *Making Wicked Problems Governable? The Case for Managed Networks in Healthcare*, Oxford University Press, Oxford.

6 Locock, L., Dopson, S., Chambers, D. and Gabbay, J. (2001) Understanding the role of opinion leaders in improving clinical effectiveness. *Social Science & Medicine*, **53**, 745–757.

7 Flodgren, G., Parmelli, E., Doumit, G. *et al* (2011) Local opinion leaders: effects on professional practice and health care outcomes. *Cochrane Database of Systematic Reviews* 2011, (2).

8 Michie, S., van Stralen, M.M. and West, R. (2011) The behaviour change wheel: a new method for characterising and designing behaviour change interventions. *Implementation Science*, **6**, 42.

9 Baker, R., Camosso-Stefinovic, J., Gillies, C. *et al.* (2010) Tailored interventions to overcome identified barriers to change: effects on professional practice and health care outcomes. *Cochrane Database of Systematic Reviews 2010*, (3).

10 Ivers, N., Jamtvedt, G., Flottorp, S. *et al* (2012) Audit and feedback: effects on professional practice and health care outcomes. *Cochrane Database of Systematic Reviews 2012*, (3).

11 Farmer, A.P., Legare, F., Turcot, L. *et al.* (2008) Printed educational materials: effects on professional practice and health care outcomes. *Cochrane Database of Systematic Reviews 2008*, (3).

12 O'Brien, M.A., Rogers, S., Jamtvedt, G. *et al.* (2007) Educational outreach visits: effects on professional practice and health care outcomes. *Cochrane Database of Systematic Reviews 2007*, (4).

13 Forsetlund, L., Bjørndal, A., Rashidian, A. *et al.* (2009) Continuing education meetings and workshops: effects on professional practice and health care outcomes. *Cochrane Database of Systematic Reviews 2009*, (2).

14 Robertson, R. and Jochelson, K. (2006) *Interventions That Change Clinician Behaviour: Mapping the Literature, The King's Fund Publication for NICE*, London.

Further reading

Grol, R., Wensing, M. and Eccles, M. (2005) *Improving Patient Care*, Elsevier, Edinburgh.

Example in Practice

Changing behaviour in primary care to improve the management of children with feverish illness

A large teaching GP practice in Hertfordshire set out to improve the quality of care for children presenting with febrile illness. The overall goal was to ensure that 95% of children under the age of five presenting with a febrile illness were assessed in accordance with the NICE guidelines. The project used the principles of improvement science to make it easier for clinicians to do the right thing and harder to do the wrong thing.

> A simple effective project made successful by paying attention to engaging other clinicians and using a systematic improvement methodology.

Source: Dr Paresh Dawda, GP.

Four key components not being measured

Children frequently present to general practice with an acute febrile illness, but despite this, studies have shown that half of the children with a serious febrile illness are not identified at first presentation.

GPs have a challenging task to identify those children with a serious illness from a large number of children who will have minor illnesses that are often self-limiting.

In order to improve the situation, NICE published guidance in 2007 (updated 2013) on the assessment and initial management of children who were less than 5 years with febrile illness.

A baseline assessment carried out at the practice revealed that the four components of the NICE-recommended clinical assessment were not happening. Temperature was recorded just over 80% of the time, capillary refill time recorded for just 30% of children, respiratory rate for fewer than 20% of children and none of the children had their heart rate measured.

Provide prompts to change current practice following education

Staff questionnaires, direct observation and *leadership walk arounds* identified a range of potential solutions in addition to the need for greater education and training. This was provided by an online learning tool, supported by NICE.

Information on normal temperature values was placed on mouse mats specifically designed with a picture of a little girl having her temperature checked to further provide a memory prompt to check the temperature. A further reminder prompt was a sticker of the same little girl below the LCD screen of tympanic thermometers.

A data entry template was created on the clinical system to capture coded data. An electronic algorithm was also created on the clinical system (EMIS LV), so that if a code was entered for a child that would suggest a condition with a fever, the computer system would check to see if the four items had been recorded and if not it would create a *forcing* function reminding the clinician to conduct these components of the assessment.

Measuring improvement

Uptake of the NICE guidelines was monitored using another tool from improvement science (known as *statistical process control chart*). Each patient was given a score of 1, 2, 3 or 4 depending on how many components of the assessment they had conducted. Each patient was then plotted on the statistical process control (SPC) chart, and the chart was annotated with the interventions.

This is an ongoing project but the actions carried out so far have clearly demonstrated that the interventions are leading to an improvement in care.

Using financial systems to support improved care

CHAPTER 5

Jennifer Field

Health Education England, Leeds, UK

Introduction

This chapter presents the issues that funders and service providers may wish to consider regarding financial systems and levers to support improved care. It is important that these are considered in the light of local circumstances as there are often different ways of achieving the same outcome, and there is no one right answer.

Most guidance is discretionary rather than mandatory, so to bring about implementation it is important to identify levers that can encourage change. Often lack of resources is cited as a barrier to improving quality. Therefore, consideration of the resources involved in a systematic, objective way is an important step in moving implementation forward. Where there is general reluctance to change, using financial incentives to encourage implementation may be useful. The evidence base for this is reviewed, following a general section on the importance of good financial management.

Consideration of financial implications and payment systems cannot be done in isolation. Often clinicians wanting to improve quality are viewed suspiciously as wanting to increase costs, whereas change driven by finance departments is viewed with suspicion from clinicians as only being motivated by saving money. Examples of payment schemes to incentivise best practice in primary care and secondary care are presented.

Best practice indicates that clinicians and finance colleagues working collaboratively together can identify solutions and build a better business case to implement evidence-based guidance and improve quality.

Achieving High Quality Care: Practical Experience from NICE, First Edition.
Edited by Gillian Leng, Val Moore and Sasha Abraham.

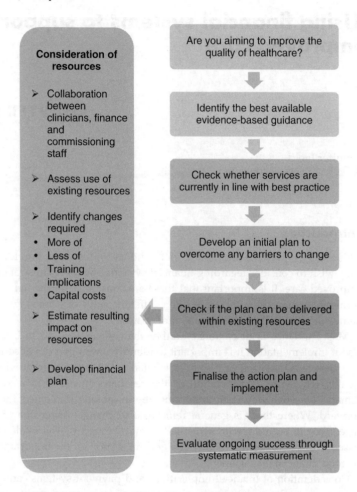

Consideration of resources

➤ Collaboration between clinicians, finance and commissioning staff

➤ Assess use of existing resources

➤ Identify changes required
• More of
• Less of
• Training implications
• Capital costs

➤ Estimate resulting impact on resources

➤ Develop financial plan

Are you aiming to improve the quality of healthcare?

Identify the best available evidence-based guidance

Check whether services are currently in line with best practice

Develop an initial plan to overcome any barriers to change

Check if the plan can be delivered within existing resources

Finalise the action plan and implement

Evaluate ongoing success through systematic measurement

Fig. 5.1 Resource considerations for achieving high-quality care.

Figure 5.1 shows where financial aspects fit within the overall process for improvement and highlight key considerations for resources.

Why is good financial management important?

The 2011 survey of challenges to implementing NICE guidance (Figure 1.2) indicates that lack of money was considered an important barrier, and 41% of respondents were concerned about resource utilisation (including resources for training/new skills and new services or equipment). A study by the Audit Commission in England found that while funding was perceived as the biggest barrier to the implementation of NICE guidance, the most significant issue they identified was weaknesses in local financial management arrangements [1, 2]. Their recommendations for improving financial management and thereby overcoming some of the barriers included developing a robust business case incorporating an assessment of the costs and savings associated with guidance; incorporating guidance implementation into financial plans; and ongoing monitoring of costs and savings arising from implementation.

Can financial systems and levers help drive improvements in the provision of health care?

A review of evidence regarding the impact of financial incentives used in changing health care professional behaviours and patient outcomes led to the conclusion that financial incentives may be effective in changing practice, but noted that the evidence has serious methodological limitations and is limited in completeness and generalisability [3].

Other research into the impact of incentives notes that some people respond to non-monetary incentives such as public service motivation or professionalism, so financial incentives should be considered alongside other motivating factors. While individuals may respond to financial incentives in the short term, incentives may be negative reinforcers in the long run, as they may conflict with intrinsic motivation by signalling to the individual that they are not trusted to perform in the absence of inducements [4]. The research evidence shows an inconsistent association between cost and health care quality, and where there is a positive association, it is only modest [5].

There is a greater body of literature that highlights the often significant costs of poor quality. This includes the direct costs of adverse events such as greater intensity of intervention required to correct mistakes, extended length of stay where patients acquire infections and complications secondary to their main condition, and more complex and lengthy follow-up that could result from poor care, not to mention potential costs of litigation. Even administrative errors can lead to considerable waste such as patients failing to attend scheduled appointments, delays in test result reporting or loss of medical records leading to repeat testing or a delay in starting treatment [6].

The inconclusive evidence does not mean that financial systems and levers are of no use, but that people designing and using them should consider how costs and effects could be monitored to aid further research in this area. This includes measuring other factors that might influence or confound the size of the effect and enabling comparisons of the cost-effectiveness of different types of incentives.

One important softer effect that has been noted is that financial incentive schemes can be useful in ensuring that quality is on the agenda in contract discussions and at board level in organisations.

How is quality incentivised in the English NHS?

The NHS is financed mainly by general taxation and is free to users at the point of delivery. Within England, there are a number of different frameworks for paying for health care services – some of which include incentives to drive quality improvements. There has also been encouragement for local schemes that reward quality improvements targeted at local priorities.

What is the QOF?

Primary care activity undertaken by general practitioners has been subject to a voluntary *Quality and Outcomes Framework* (QOF) scheme since 2004, which rewards them for how well they care for patients. The QOF contains groups of indicators, against which practices score points according to their level of achievement. Put simply, the higher the score, the higher the financial reward for the practice. The design of incentives for the QOF has sometimes followed a phased approach, whereby the initial indicator rewards the identification of patients with a disease or condition. Following this, there may be an additional or amended indicator that rewards a process known to be linked to improved outcomes, and, finally, the indicator may require achievement of more detailed targets. For example, establishing a register of all patients with diabetes, before then being rewarded for undertaking regular monitoring of HbA1c levels for patients on the register, and the latest iteration of QOF requires achieving a specific target level of HbA1c in a certain percentage of their patients in the preceding period. Trying to introduce a challenging target level of HbA1c in the majority of patients without first incentivising data collection and routine monitoring may not have been so readily accepted if introduced in one step.

What are PbR and BPT?

Secondary care activity undertaken by acute hospitals has been subject to the *Payment by Results* (PbR) initiative – a national framework for reimbursing a significant proportion of activity in acute hospitals. In

2011–2012, PbR represented over 60% of acute hospital income and about one-third of commissioning budgets [7]. It was introduced with the initial objective of supporting increased capacity and reduced waiting times; however, it has evolved to be both a way of containing prices and, more recently, also aims to reward quality through the introduction of best practice tariffs (BPT).

BPTs have been structured and priced to encourage patient care that is both high quality and cost effective. These are discussed in more detail later in this chapter. BPT represents a major change to the current tariff structure that is based on national average costs of activity. There is consistency between BPTs and NICE guidance recommendations, where relevant.

PbR in combination with patient level costing enables questions such as 'patient X's treatment costs 50% more than the revenue that was earned – why?' to be asked. These are far more powerful questions than 'why was your budget overspent by 10% this month?'. Looking at costs at the patient level is easy for clinicians to understand and better ways of doing this are being developed.

What is CQUIN?

Commissioning for Quality and Innovation (CQUIN) started in 2009–2010 as a payment framework to reward excellence by linking a proportion of providers' income to the achievement of local quality improvement goals, and has also included some national goals such as identification of patients with dementia and patient safety issues. Research has focused on BPT, but when compared with the experience of CQUIN, it has been found that CQUIN measures were less likely to be based on evidence but subject to greater negotiation and executive attention [8].

To end this section, the following case study is instructive of the benefits and the potentially unintended consequences of financial incentives.

The introduction of a BPT for fragility hip fracture as outlined in Box 5.1 is facilitated by there being a nationally accepted method for collecting data through the hip fracture database. Most hospitals were already regularly submitting data to this database, so no additional administrative burden is placed on providers. This database has been a valuable research tool for a number of organisations including Nottingham University where researchers found that the proportion of patients being operated on promptly increased from 57.8% in 2007–2008 to 70.0% in 2010–2011. There was also a reduction in the proportion of patients who died within 30 days of admission from

Box 5.1 A national level incentive scheme to improve hip fracture care

One BPT covers best practice in the management of patients with fragility hip fracture. This is a common reason for admission to hospital with about 70 000–75 000 hip fractures occurring in England each year, and as this condition is associated with ageing it is predicted to rise. The tariff is an additional payment on top of the base tariff price if all of the best practice compliance criteria are met in patients aged over 60 admitted non-electively for fragility hip fracture. The criteria are based on evidence and the NICE guideline recommendations that are readily measurable and are as follows:
- Time to surgery within 36 h from arrival in an emergency department, or time of diagnosis of an inpatient, to the start of anaesthesia
- Admitted under the joint care of a consultant geriatrician and a consultant orthopaedic surgeon
- Admitted using an assessment protocol agreed by geriatric medicine, orthopaedic surgery and anaesthesia
- Assessed by a geriatrician in the perioperative period (within 72 h of admission)
- Postoperative geriatrician-directed multiprofessional rehabilitation team
- Fracture prevention assessments (falls and bone health).

7.0% to 6.1% over the same period [8]. Therefore, although most of the incentivised criteria relate to process, they are having an effect on outcomes and reducing avoidable deaths.

One unintended consequence of the introduction of the BPT is that the proportion of patients undergoing surgery within 48 hours has fallen, perhaps because a focus on meeting the 36 hours target has been detrimental to those patients who go beyond 36 hours. A similar effect has been noted with the stroke BPT requirement to scan patients within 24 hours of admission. If there are capacity issues and a patient has breached 24 hours, there is an incentive to use the next available slot to prevent another patient breaching 24 hours, thereby lengthening the delay for the original patient.

How can funding arrangements incorporate NICE and other evidence-based guidance?

Planning and funding care involve a number of aspects, including the following:
- Assessing the needs of the population served
- Reviewing current service provision and identifying gaps or over-provision
- Decisions about priorities
- Specification of services

- Securing appropriate services
- Managing demand while ensuring appropriate access
- Managing performance (delivery, quality and outcomes)

Underpinning all of the above is a requirement to work within the resources available, which often means decisions about priorities become challenging when the cost of meeting the identified need exceeds the resources available. When there is growth in the health care budget, decisions tend to focus on where to invest additional resources. When there is limited growth in the budget, perhaps combined with rising demand driven by an ageing population, new technologies and treatments, financial management is more challenging. This requires the total budget available and outcomes achieved to be considered, not just the incremental increases in budget and demand. This will inevitably lead to re-prioritisation involving disinvestment in some activities to free up resources for re-investment in areas considered a higher priority.

Using evidence-based guidance can help funding decisions through providing robust evidence-based recommendations about clinically effective and cost-effective treatments and interventions to underpin decisions where there are competing priorities. Often guidance will identify where early diagnosis and intervention can deliver improved patient outcomes and avoid the need for more complex and costly treatment in the future. This is particularly true of public health recommendations, which frequently focus on prevention.

The implementation of evidence-based recommendations requires an initial assessment of the likely financial implications of any change – tools are available alongside NICE guidance to support this process. Information about incidence and prevalence of disease is a useful starting point when assessing need or considering thresholds for treatment.

Where appropriate, the whole health care system needs to be considered, such as where a care pathway involves multiple providers with transitions between primary care and secondary care, or jointly working between sectors such as acute and mental health or community providers.

What are the components of a good business case?

Business cases are one means of obtaining authority to invest in making change. The scale of the change is likely to determine the level of authority required. Producing a good business case should be proportionate to the proposed change. For example, the business case for a major service reconfiguration involving multiple sites across a health economy should be longer and more detailed than a project that impacts at an individual ward level.

Irrespective of the scale of the change there are a number of components that good business cases contain. This includes information on the following:

- The nature of the proposed change – what is included or excluded.
- The population affected by the change.
- How the business case fits with the strategic direction for improving services.
- The measurable outcomes to be achieved.
- How the proposal represents value for money.
- Any non-recurrent investment required to enable change.
- Any recurrent annual increase in service delivery cost.
- Whether the initiative will release resources or efficiencies.
- Evidence of effectiveness.
- Risks and mitigating actions.

Business cases for larger projects may include additional information including an options appraisal, sensitivity analysis and project management arrangements for delivery. An often forgotten element of business development is post-change review to check whether the change delivered the anticipated benefits at the anticipated cost. Undertaking this can provide important learning points for future business case development.

Why should finance be considered across a health economy?

It may be that while good quality will deliver cost savings, the financial system – particularly where there is more than one organisation involved – removes or reduces the incentive for the health care provider to deliver best quality care. For example, stopping smoking prior to an elective procedure is proven to result in less complications [9]; however, the tariff is structured such that a health care provider is frequently paid a higher amount should a patient having an elective procedure be subject to complications; therefore, there is no financial incentive for the health care provider to encourage smoking cessation prior to surgery.

Similarly, for other public health interventions, the health care provider might use additional resources to encourage increased physical activity, but the savings arising from improved levels of fitness such as the reduced risk of future cardiovascular events will not benefit the provider to whom reduced activity may mean reduced income. It then falls to those with a view of the whole system to take a more holistic whole systems view and look at whether and how certain behaviours can be incentivised.

In addition to positive incentives of additional income to reward good quality care, some financial systems can also have negative incentives or penalties for poor quality care. An example of this includes the fines that English hospitals may face if they do not meet targets for reducing the incidence of the hospital acquired infection *Clostridium difficile*, or recent developments in PbR so that readmissions within 30 days of discharge will not be paid for unless it can be demonstrated that they were not the fault of the provider.

While no payment for readmissions is a worthy aim, there have been considerable difficulties in developing a scheme that is robust and does not unfairly penalise providers for unrelated admissions. For example, if someone who had a successful elective procedure had an unrelated car accident within 30 days of discharge, then it is unfair to withhold payment for the car accident admission. Even patients that are frequently in and out of hospital may be outside the control of the provider in that readmissions could be as a result of negligence by the patient or a lack of community care facilities rather than poor care from the provider. However, the potential loss of income does encourage acute providers to challenge those responsible for community care and primary care to provide good follow-up and avoid readmissions where possible.

Summary

Considering financial incentives and funding flows is an important step in achieving high-quality health care. Indeed some research indicates that good quality care costs less than providing poor quality care, and this in itself should be an incentive to improve quality.

Financial management arrangements should be integrated into the main business and management arrangements of organisations, and these should all be aligned to the objective of achieving quality improvement. The whole system, including financial management, has a part to play in assisting rather than hindering quality improvement as well as specific financial incentive schemes. Developing a robust business case that includes non-financial information will be key to this. As discussed earlier, having clinical and financial colleagues all working together to develop the business case may result in a more solid case that has wider stakeholder buy-in.

In order to be most effective, financial incentive schemes must be well designed to incentivise the right action and not to introduce unintended consequences. For financial incentive schemes to work, they should be based on evidence and data that are credible, valid and reliable and ideally do not add any administrative burden through using existing data flows to reward achievement in a timely manner.

Learning from practice

1 It is possible to create financial incentives to improve quality, but these need to be carefully designed.
2 Incentives can be either positive or negative – rewarding improvement or penalising quality failures.
3 The impact on both the provider of care and those funding care needs to be considered. Often something that is beneficial across the health economy could disadvantage one party financially.
4 Irrespective of whether quality improvement is incentivised, it can avoid the high costs (including financial and reputational) of poor quality.
5 There needs to be a clear link between what is measured and incentivised and anticipated improved outcomes.
6 The administrative burden and what can easily be measured need to be considered when developing incentive schemes.

References

1 Audit Commission (2005) *Managing the Financial Implications of NICE Gudiance*, Audit Commission, London.
2 Audit Commission (2012) *Best Practice Tariffs and Their Impact*, Audit Commission, London.
3 Flodgren, G., Eccles, M.P., Shepperd, S. *et al.* (2011) An overview of reviews evaluating the effectiveness of financial incentives in changing healthcare professional behaviours and patient outcomes. *The Cochrane Collaboration.*
4 McDonald, R. and Cheraghi-Sohi, S. (2010) *The Impact of Incentives on the Behaviour and Performance of Primary Care Professionals*, Queen's Printer and Controller of HMSO, London.
5 Hussey, P.S., Wertheimer, S. and Mehrotra, A.A. (2013) The association between health care quality and cost: a systematic review. *Annals of Internal Medicine*, **158** (1), 27–34.
6 Øvretveit, D.J. (2009) *Does improving quality save money?*, The Health Foundation, London.
7 Department of Health (2011) *A Simple Guide to Payment by Results*, Department of Health, Leeds.
8 Ruth McDonald, S.Z. (2012) *A Qualitative and Quantitative Evaluation of the Introduction of Best Practice Tariffs*, Nottingham University, Nottingham.
9 Theadom, A. and Cropley, M. (2006) Effects of preoperative smoking cessation on the incidence and risk of intraoperative and postoperative complications in adult smokers: a systematic review. *Tobacco Control*, **15**, 352–358.

Further reading

NICE (2011) *Assessing Cost Impact – Methods Guide*, NICE, London.

Payment by results commentary, http://www.kingsfund.org.uk/publications /payment-results-0 (accessed 10 April 2014).

Example in Practice

Building a business case: to redesign diabetes services

Services for patients with diabetes in the Midlands were redesigned based on NICE guidance.

A multidisciplinary team (MDT) of clinicians was created to manage the support and services required. The MDT was funded through savings made using NICE-recommended human insulin for treatment, as opposed to analogue insulin.

> An increase in the use of NICE-recommended human insulin resulted in savings of more than £600,000.

> Source: Sue Smith, Head of Prescribing and Medicines Management.

Remodelling services for type 2 diabetes

Information from a variety of sources suggested that services offered for type 2 diabetes could be improved in the Midlands. The aim was to redesign these services so that they could provide greater consistency of care and reduce dependency on treatment in secondary care.

A clinical reference group (CRG) was set up to design and deliver a new best practice model of care, providing information, support and care to patients so they could make informed choices about their conditions.

The CRG identified the creation of an MDT to manage the support and services associated with diabetes, as a priority action. It drew up a *wish list* of all the services and types of professionals that an MDT might include such as consultants, specialist nurses, podiatrists, dietetics, services for psychological support and ways of providing care closer to the homes of patients.

However, the group soon realised that there would be no extra funding available to resource such a team, and that existing resources would have to be used differently. In order to overcome the problem, it took recommendations from NICE's guidance on type 2 diabetes and came up with a novel method of generating the income required to fund the MDT.

Using savings from implementing NICE guidance to redesign services

The CRG observed that current treatment with insulin in the Midlands contrasted with NICE guidance. NICE recommends that treatment should begin with human NPH insulin, and that this should be taken at bedtime or twice daily according to need.

Yet the CRG found that treatment with human NPH insulin only accounted for 15% of the total amount of long and intermediate acting insulin used; almost the opposite of what would be expected if NICE guidance was being followed.

The group identified that the first-line use of analogue insulin costs an estimated additional £1 million per year in the area. In addition, an audit of practice nurses found that the majority had only received training in implementing analogue insulin.

It consequently set up a 1-day training course for practice nurses run by diabetes specialist nurses and a medicines management pharmacist. This course runs every 6–8 weeks on an ongoing basis and explains the practical aspects of initiating human NPH insulin and the evidence base behind its use.

Multidisciplinary team brought several improvements

When the course started in September 2010, human insulin accounted for 15% of all long and intermediate acting insulin.

By July 2012, this had grown to 25%, resulting in savings of more than £600 000.

These savings were used to fund the MDT, which in turn has achieved the following improvements.

These include a 48% reduction in admissions, which has resulted in savings of £301 000, mentoring and support for primary care clinicians to avoid unnecessary referrals integrated working, and the use of *diabetes specialist workers* to support hard to reach patient groups.

The MDT has also implemented greater integrated working, with 55 primary care practices and clinics involving a range of specialists, including a consultant diabetologist.

Learning from practice

- It is important and helpful for clinicians to see that the savings made from following NICE guidelines were ring-fenced and reinvested in diabetes services.
- A MDT is crucial and has a huge impact on service design.

Using measurement to support change and improvements in health care

CHAPTER 6

Nick Baillie

Indicators, Health and Social Care Quality Team, National Institute for Health and Care Excellence, Manchester, UK

Introduction

Previous chapters have described the principles of guidance development, some of the characteristics of health systems and organisations that are needed to influence change, and the process of change. In this chapter, we will look at the role of data and measurement in relation to change in three potential roles: stimulating change, confirming that change has been made and sustaining change.

Firstly, the availability of data and measures can in itself be something that stimulates and leads to change. By developing and routinely reporting on measures of quality, focus can be brought to important issues and thus initiate positive changes. We will therefore consider whether measurement can be a core component of change programmes in its own right.

Secondly, in the context of the processes of change described in the rest of this book, data and measures can be used to determine whether the aims set for improvement at the start of any project have been met. Evaluation through routine data and measurement is therefore an important consideration in the process of guidance implementation, and one of the final pieces in the jigsaw.

Thirdly, there is a need to think about how we sustain changes that have been made, and the role of routine data and measurement. A lot of effort is often put into making initial changes happen. It is therefore worthwhile

Achieving High Quality Care: Practical Experience from NICE, First Edition.
Edited by Gillian Leng, Val Moore and Sasha Abraham.
© 2014 John Wiley & Sons, Ltd. Published 2014 by John Wiley & Sons, Ltd.

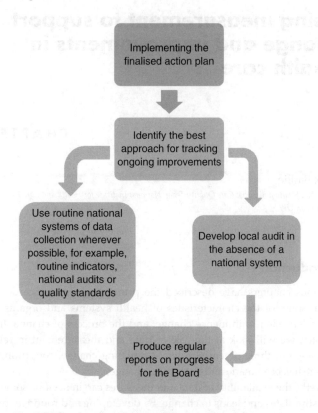

Fig. 6.1 How to sustain high-quality care through measurement.

making sure that when the initial focus and enthusiasm have died down, changes are sustained.

This chapter therefore seeks to illustrate some of the key factors that those working in quality improvement may want to consider in terms of routine measurement and data collection, and how measurement can help implementation projects, help their evaluation and help sustain changes that have been made (Figure 6.1). Experience from the work of NICE and case studies are used to illustrate the theory and demonstrate how the momentum of change can be maintained in terms of the following:

- Developing routine measures
- Reporting and communicating data
- Leadership for sustaining change

How can measurement be used to support change?

Developing measures and indicators: lessons from the national experience

An important part of the process of change is to consider whether regular reports and data about practice can inspire change, help to establish whether projects have been successful and ensure improvements are sustained when this focus is removed. One of the primary ways this can be achieved, and the focus of this chapter, is by setting up systems that provide regular feedback and reports on progress. This helps to bring a focus on, and understanding of, current practice and any changes that have been made. This type of approach is grounded in approaches to change such as audit and feedback, which we know can be effective ways to achieve change [1]. There are similarities between using routine measures and audit and feedback – we know re-audit is an important part of quality improvement, and that it is best to provide feedback on a frequent basis.

Working at a national level, NICE recognises the importance of routine measurement as part of the process of maintaining change. While efforts are made to provide tools and support for local use as highlighted in Chapter 4, there is now an increasing focus on building associated measures into routinely collected data sets. Routine data can provide a starting point for local quality improvement, but some standard definitions in numerator and denominators may need to be adapted to reflect local circumstances (see Box 6.1).

This approach of using nationally set measures and indicators could, and should, be mirrored as part of local implementation and change projects: clinical teams should consider information and measures that will help them track progress on an ongoing basis, and how information

Box 6.1 Hip fracture guideline: example quality measure

Statement: People with hip fracture have surgery on the day of, or the day after, admission
    Quality measure: Proportion of people with hip fracture who receive surgery on the day of, or the day after, admission.
    Numerator: The number of people in the denominator who receive surgery on the day of, or the day after, admission.
    Denominator: The number of people with hip fracture having surgery.

teams can help build this into systems that provide regular feedback. Those focusing on service redesign should consider what the key markers of success are and how this can be measured through data routinely collected by those providing the service and reported at regular intervals.

There are, however, a number of further lessons from the NICE experience that also warrant consideration when translated to the local level. Table 6.1 describes broad, high-level quality measures and formal indicators. It is important that the difference between these is acknowledged and related to how they are to be used. Table 6.1 provides a summary of this in the context of quality measures and indicators developed by NICE in relation to quality standards. This may provide food for thought at a local level where measures need to be designed in the absence of a national measure.

Box 6.2 Use of quality measures to improve stroke services

A London Provider Service reviewed the NICE stroke guideline in order to decide which would apply to the local rehabilitation service. Four of the recommendations were immediately seen to be relevant, and two others added after discussion on their implications for practice. An example of one of the quality statements and measures included is as follows.

Statement: Patients with stroke are offered a minimum of 45 min of each active therapy that is required, for a minimum of 5 days a week, at a level that enables the patient to meet their rehabilitation goals for as long as they are continuing to benefit from the therapy and are able to tolerate it.

Quality measure: Proportion of patients with stroke who are offered 45 min of each active therapy that is required, for as long as they are continuing to benefit from the therapy and are able to tolerate it.

Numerator: The number of patients who are offered a minimum of 45 min of each active therapy for a minimum of 5 days a week.

Denominator: The number of patients with a new stroke episode in hospital.

Data on the agreed measures have been collected for the first three quarters of the 2011–2012 financial year. Most data showed that achievement against the measures continued to rise throughout the year with the biggest improvements noted in patients being allocated key workers to act as a central point of contact and patients having access to all appropriate therapies (quarter 3 data shows that 91% patients are receiving physiotherapy, 90% occupational health and 76% speech and language therapy for 45 minutes a day, 5 days a week). These have been incorporated into metrics and targets for the service that are being reported to local commissioners as performance data.

Table 6.1 Comparison of NICE quality measures and indicators

	Quality measures	Formal indicators
Characteristics	• Broad definitions • Additional definitions may be needed and can be adapted for local use • Not piloted or tested	• Highly defined and reproducible • Cannot be adapted and definitions should be followed • Tested as part of development process
Use	• Provide a focus for local quality improvement activity	• Provide a focus for local or national quality improvement activity • Provide a mechanism for comparison

Developing measures and indicators: issues for local consideration

The use of quality measures and indicators can be an effective, low-resource mechanism for obtaining feedback when they are part of routine data collection. However, their use and purpose need to be differentiated. In terms of measurement, there are often concepts that differ slightly at regional, organisational, team and individual levels. Where the focus is purely on delivering quality improvement internally within a single organisation, the differences do not necessarily matter. However, where there is to be some sort of comparison, even if it is purely for benchmarking purposes, there is a need to ensure that apples are being compared with apples, and pears compared with pears.

The use of indicators and standard definitions has the benefit of bringing consistency longitudinally and between organisations, teams and individuals. This brings improved ability to benchmark between services and measure change more accurately over time. Both quality measures and indicators can therefore be used to support quality improvement, but it is only indicators that should be used for comparison.

There are a number of further considerations from the NICE experience in terms of developing indicators for regular measurement. Where data are to be collected regularly and fed back, they can lead to unintended consequences – these may occur where the focus of the measurement distorts what is intended to be the true action or outcome. For example, there may be alternative behaviours that can lead to improvements in the subject of the measurement, or the focus on one particular area leads to knock-on effects and negative impacts in other parts of the system. For these reasons, NICE includes a testing process as part of the development of indicators – similarly, at a local level, it may be important to include an evaluation of unintended consequences as part of any regular measurement plan.

It is also important to consider how patients can be involved in aspects of routine measurement, and NICE reflects this in its processes of developing measures and indicators. There are a number of key ways in which the patient's perspective can be important. First, patients can help to define the key improvements that are being planned to ensure that they are focused on delivering the most important outcomes. Second, the patient's perspective can also be helpful in evaluating whether there are any unintended consequences that the focus on measurement may bring, as they will often be the first to feel the impact. The third way in which patient involvement is important is in considering whether any elements of patient experience could routinely be collected to complement more clinically focused measures. This is particularly important to ensure that patient's feedback correlates with any changes in clinical practice, and again can be important indication of any unintended consequences. Finally, it can be important to involve patients in the general leadership, as they can be influential and an important lever for change (this is discussed more in the following section).

What is the best way to report and communicate data?

In the previous section of this chapter, the role of measurement in sustaining change has been highlighted and likened to the process of audit and feedback. If the development of routine measures and indicators is the *audit* part of this process, then we also need to consider the *feedback* part of the process and the principles of how best to communicate about practice on an ongoing basis.

Involving the team

The first question to consider should probably be to whom measures and indicators should be reported? The most obvious group are the staff involved in delivering the practice being measured. There are a number of important reasons to include this group, not least because they can help to validate data and to identify anomalies before anything is shared more widely. This is important, particularly in the early stages of developing indicators.

To help sustain change, it is important that staff are involved in developing plans and responding to any key messages within the data. These messages will be important to communicate alongside the data to other audiences, and this should happen early on in the process. It is important to celebrate success with staff, and not just focus on the areas where further change is needed. If the point of the exercise is to sustain change, improvement needs to be recognised and rewarded as appropriate.

Reporting to the board

The people at board level in any health care organisation are ultimately responsible for the quality of care, and are therefore a key audience for information about the ongoing success of any change. This not only helps in terms of accountability but also ensures that success can be acknowledged at the most senior level in an organisation. Where additional action is needed to sustain change, communication at this level also ensures high-level ongoing support. Finally, by presenting data at board level through a simple reporting mechanism, focus and attention will be maintained on a particular area to help maintain progress.

Engaging patients through reporting of data

Patients, users of services and their carers are also important audiences for data and measures about change and quality of services. This is partly because of the benefits of being publicly accountable for care, as well as seeking to generally improve quality and maintain change. Reporting to patients and carers, particularly where an initial improvement has been achieved, also helps to develop expectations of the future level of service. This group can then help to prompt, question and ask for a particular level of service, thus helping the change to be sustained and become part of normal everyday practice.

Formats for reporting to each audience

Having given consideration to the audiences, thought should also be given to different formats and mediums for communicating data about change. In the early stages of presenting data, a two-way dialogue is probably needed between those with the informatics expertise and the audience. Discussion in forums such as team meetings or public board meetings can be helpful in identifying inaccurate data,

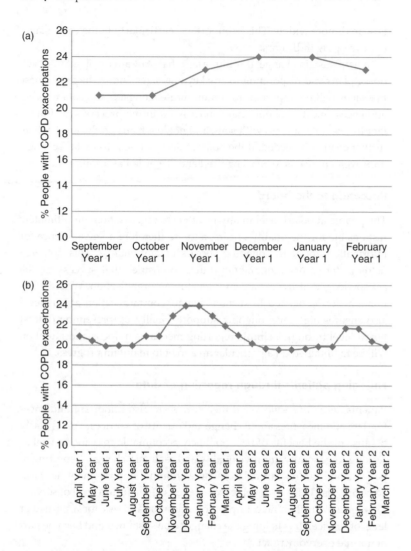

Fig. 6.2 Charts showing proportion of people with COPD suffering exacerbations indicative of typical patterns.

understanding unintended consequences, celebrating success and establishing responses. However, perhaps one of the most important issues at this stage is ensuring that data are understood. Using data in more open and transparent ways can lead to risks in terms of misinterpretation.

The two charts in Figure 6.2 show the proportion of patients with chronic obstructive pulmonary disease (COPD) suffering exacerbations.

Figure 6.2a shows data from the early stages of a measurement project to improve the care of people with COPD after 6 months. It suggests that there could be a concern that there is an upwards trend, and that perhaps patients with COPD may not be receiving the best care possible from the organisation. However, Figure 6.2b shows the same data but for an extended period over the following 18 months. This chart suggests that there is generally a downwards trend in people with COPD suffering exacerbations. This highlights the importance of considering how much data are needed to identify a trend in any measurement project, and the influence of external factors such as seasonal variation.

The importance therefore, particularly in the early stages of engagement with informatics experts to ensure that data are presented and interpreted accurately, is vital. Over time, as users become more familiar with the data, it may be possible to move towards less intensive engagement and written reports, as staff, patients and carers become able to access data at the same time on organisations' websites.

How to provide leadership for change?

There is a large evidence base that supports the need for leadership in the process of managing change. Although much of this evidence relates to the time-limited act of stimulating change, the same lessons can be applied to the ongoing process of evaluating improvement or sustaining change through use of data and regular measurement [2].

Acknowledging the structure and context of service provision

Before considering questions about which specific individuals to involve in sustaining change, it is important to acknowledge the structural context. Change often focuses around those involved in the operational day-to-day provision of services, but ongoing support can also come from those managing and funding the service – they can have an important influence on the type of data that are collected. The role that managers and funders play in maintaining change is also essential: contracts need to be updated to reflect changes; effects on parallel, upstream or downstream services need to be managed; the focus needs to be maintained in a way that does not absorb huge amounts of time.

Simple ways to do this include building measures for quality improvement into any contracts or service specifications with providers of health care. Focusing on areas that have been identified as important for quality improvement, the measures should define numerators and denominators that are relevant locally. Managers and funders should therefore be considered as one of the key players in sustaining and maintaining change, even where the primary drive and focus may be coming from a service provider.

Identifying the individual or groups to provide feedback

There are further lessons from the experience of audit and feedback that relate to the use of routine data and indicators. The evidence shows that feedback is an effective approach in generating change, but there are important contextual considerations. There appears to be a significantly bigger improvement where feedback is delivered by a supervisor or senior colleague, indicating the need for those at most senior levels to maintain their enthusiasm to support sustainable change.

It is important to be aware that, although there is a natural tendency to engage with those who have a positive approach to measurement and change, there is also a need to engage with those who may not be so positive. This need is perhaps greater in the context of sustaining change than the initial stages of establishing the change. It is when focus drops that there is a higher risk of returning to former practice, and therefore those who are generally less positive need to be actively engaged.

Finally, it is important to remember that patients can be very influential in the process. They have an important role in helping to determine measures and indicators, and should also be part of the team that regularly reviews feedback from routine data collection (for example, Box 6.3).

Box 6.3 QIPP safe care: the NHS Safety Thermometer

The NHS Safety Thermometer is designed to provide a quick and simple method for surveying patient harms at the point of care, analysing results at a local level and a national level. The aim is to raise awareness, stimulate action and monitor improvements over time. The tool measures four types of harm: pressure ulcers, falls, urinary infection (in patients with catheters) and venous thromboembolism.

A multidisciplinary expert group was established to agree the measures to be used and these were then put through a testing process using a Plan, Do, Study, Act (PDSA) methodology. The focus of the tool is on stimulating improvement at a local level and over 160 originations engaged in a large-scale pilot process including patients in acute, community and residential care settings as well as in their own homes.

The purpose of the development and testing process was to
- agree and refine operational definitions for the measures;
- modify the data collection tool/survey based on feedback;
- agree sampling and data collection methods and how data should be interpreted;
- engage front line teams in data collection at the point of care.

As a result of this process, a set of measures were agreed that could be defined and used in a similar way wherever the patient is located. The survey is completed by those caring for the patient (usually nurses), which does mean there is a requirement on clinicians to input data (less than 10 min per patient). In order to reduce the burden of data collection, data are only collected on a single day each month. The sample is large enough to give statistically valid data that is representative of the overall burden of harm. The method does not tell organisations everything they need to know about harm, or count the exact number of harms, but rather acts a temperature check that can be used to measure improvement over time.

The NHS Safety Thermometer provides the clinician with the opportunity to instantly review, verify and check the data, including a comparison of changes over time.

The data can also be analysed at ward or team level with comparisons at regional and national levels. This then also provides those units where results seem to be particularly high or low with a second opportunity to verify their data, as well as the chance to consider action plans. In terms of the latter, there is a need to think about how data are interpreted and avoid knee jerk reactions to high or low results that may just be due to natural fluctuations in the data. Guidance is therefore provided on the interpretation of results, and analytical techniques such as run and control charts are used. Guidance does state that NHS Safety Thermometer data should be triangulated with data from other sources, such as incident reporting, audit data or administrative data to give a full picture of harm.

Summary overview

This chapter has demonstrated the importance of focusing on how change can be maintained right from the outset of any quality improvement project. The three key aspects of this are using key measures derived from routine data collections wherever possible, finding ways to communicate this across key audiences and ensuring that leadership continues to be provided over time.

Learning from practice

1 Use routine data sets wherever possible to minimise the burden of data collection.
2 Consider early on how measures are intended to be used, and therefore how much rigour is needed to develop them.
3 Check whether the process of routinely measuring and feeding back on particular aspects of practice is causing unintended consequences elsewhere within the system.

4 Communicate measures on a regular basis by engaging junior and senior staff within the organisation, patients and the public, and funders and managers of the service.
5 Ensure that any data feedback and reporting are accompanied by messages that help ensure it is interpreted correctly.

References

1 Ivers N., Jamtvedt G., Flottorp S., Young J. M., Odgaard-Jensen J., French S. D., O'Brien, M. A., Johansen M., Grimshaw J., Oxman A. D. (2012) Audit and feedback: effects on professional practice and healthcare outcomes. *Cochrane Database of Systematic Reviews 2012*, Issue 6. Art. No: CD000259. 10.1002/14651858 .CD000259.pub3.
2 Flodgren G, Parmelli E, Doumit G, Gattellari M, O'Brien MA, Grimshaw J, Eccles MP (2011) Local opinion leaders: effects on professional practice and health care outcomes. *Cochrane Database of Systematic Reviews 2011*, Issue 8. Art. No.: CD000125. 10.1002/14651858.CD000125.pub4.

Further reading

The following websites may be helpful in thinking about the types of things that can be measured routinely and are currently available at a national level:
Agency for Healthcare Research and Quality, Quality Indicators http://www .qualityindicators.ahrq.gov/ (accessed 10 April 2014).
Advancing Quality Alliance http://www.advancingqualitynw.nhs.uk/index.php (accessed 10 April 2014).
Health and Social care Information Centre (HSCIC), Indicators for Quality Improvement http://www.hscic.gov.uk/iqi (accessed 10 April 2014).
NHS Quest http://www.quest.nhs.uk/ (accessed 10 April 2014).
NHS Safety Thermometer http://harmfreecare.org/measurement/nhs-safety -thermometer/ (accessed 10 April 2014).
http://www.ic.nhs.uk/thermometer (accessed 10 April 2014).

Example in Practice

Setting up a service for peripheral arterial disease in the North West of England

Poor outcomes for cardiovascular disease, an outdated service model and the need to manage resources more effectively convinced a team of clinicians in North East of England to redesign services for diagnosing, treating and managing peripheral arterial disease.

> The NICE guideline gave focus to our plans to redesign services for patients and enabled us to plan a more coherent and effective approach to the management of peripheral arterial disease.
>
> Source: Martin Fox, Vascular Specialist, Podiatrist.

Using NICE guidance to redesign services

Peripheral arterial disease (PAD) happens when arteries narrow, causing poor circulation. It mainly affects arteries taking blood to the legs. Clinicians involved in PAD in the North West of England identified it as a key risk factor in the area's high rate of cardiovascular disease (CVD) morbidity and mortality. They were frequently seeing the consequences of late diagnosis and undermanagement of PAD, resulting in avoidable amputations and vascular-related deaths, inappropriate referrals to hospital and resources being wasted. A team of vascular nurse specialists and podiatrists wanted to improve early detection and long-term management of PAD and save costs by reducing unnecessary hospital referrals. Using the NICE guideline on lower limb PAD, they commissioned a community-based service which has the following parameters:

- encouraged early referral of cases of PAD
- offered an appointment within 1 month at a choice of five locations

- carried out non-invasive, PAD assessments and diagnosis
- educated patients on CVD and the risks of not treating leg circulation disease
- worked with other teams to promote best medical therapy and healthy living (e.g. exercise and quitting smoking)
- ensured severe or deteriorating cases were referred to vascular surgeons.

Benefits of managing PAD in the community

Since setting the service up, the team has already begun to see positive results. Patient surveys have shown high levels of satisfaction with the choice of location, the prompt offer of appointments, the clinical treatment plans and the written and verbal information provided about PAD and the service. They have also developed a database to help identify the PAD population, manage PAD patients in the community and devise individual treatment plans for them, involving their GP and other community teams (best medicines, supervised exercise, stop smoking, weight management, diabetes etc.).

Learning from practice

- It is important to engage with the relevant clinical teams from a range of disciplines, before starting a redesign programme.
- Ensure the staff who deliver the service have the right level of knowledge and skills.
- The clinical diagnosis, health education and promotion and treatment for PAD are essential to effective delivery.

Overall they found that, of the patients diagnosed with PAD, 80% could be managed in the community through GP care and healthy living programmes and only 20% needed to see a vascular specialist in hospital. This has resulted in a 40% cost saving to the health and social care system and has freed up hospital resources for those who needed them more. There have also been positive trends around CVD rates in the area because more people are considering and engaging in lifestyle changes than they were before.

Conclusion and reflections

Danny Keenan[1] and Sasha Abraham[2]

[1]Department of Cardiothoracic Surgery, Manchester Heart Centre, Central Manchester University Hospitals NHS Foundation Trust, Manchester, UK
[2]Wapping Group Practice, London, UK

Introduction

We are two clinical professionals working in primary care and acute care who are associated with NICE through our participation in groups or committees. Improving the care we offer to patients has always been important. Achieving high-quality care needs several fundamental things to come together. These apply, no matter where the care is delivered, whether a massive hospital or a small general practice surgery. The first of these is to understand that everything we do is for the good of those who are ill either in front of us now or potentially in front of us in the future. The ability to have a dialogue with our patients cannot be underestimated.

This chapter consists of our conclusions and reflections on previous chapters, and builds on two themes that we think are highly important to the process of continuous improvement: clinical audit and leadership.

While the focus of previous chapters has been on improvement based on high-quality guidance, it is worth reminding readers of the implications of failure. Unfortunately in Britain, we have had a series of high-profile failures, in one form or another, in the delivery of health care. These failures have involved individual and professional failures (Ledward, Shipman, Ayling, Neale, Kerr/Haslam) and institutional failures and cross-cutting failures (the Bristol paediatric heart surgery failure, methacillin-resistant *Staphylococcus aureus* infections in hospital, dignity and nutrition in hospital). But similar types of failure can be seen in most care systems round the world [1]. The most recent of these, in England, has led to an enquiry with 290 recommendations for

Achieving High Quality Care: Practical Experience from NICE, First Edition.
Edited by Gillian Leng, Val Moore and Sasha Abraham.
© 2014 John Wiley & Sons, Ltd. Published 2014 by John Wiley & Sons, Ltd.

improvement for all concerned with the delivery of acute care. These failures have led to public frustration with the somewhat lethargic approach to the adoption of different and better ways of providing care, including basic matters of poor hygiene procedures, and spiralling costs.

In addition, there appears to be a gap between the evidence as to what should be done clinically and what actually is done [2]. We need to be able to keep on top of the current definition of clinical quality, which changes with astounding rapidity, and analyse and review our own practice repeatedly to make progress. Alongside this, the consumers of health care are, rightly, becoming increasingly sophisticated with high expectations.

Why we think high-quality evidence should be sought?

The earlier chapters have been a journey through the principles underlying how current health care systems use, or should use, the various tools available to achieve high-quality care for all and, in particular, the development of evidence-based medicine. The rationale behind the seeking out and use of best evidence remains as it was when the concept was introduced. Evidence-based medicine is the conscientious, explicit and judicious use of current best evidence in making decisions about the care of individual patients. The practice of evidence-based medicine means integrating individual clinical expertise with the best available clinical evidence from systematic research [3]. Evidence-based practice is about reducing variation in practice, not about reducing individual clinical freedom. Indeed it is more about integrating individual clinical experience with scientifically derived evidence into treatment tailored for an individual patient.

In the general practice setting, we are faced with a great number of patients with various complex medical problems. It is difficult to know how to treat every single medical condition by memory and experience. It is down to the individual doctor to keep up to date with the latest guidance and by using evidence-based medicine, such as NICE guidance that acts as an aid in treating patients. The guidance serves to act as a useful tool, drawn up through research evidence. However, through clinical experience, this guidance may not be suitable for every individual patient and is tailored accordingly by the clinician.

One problem we have is that the medical literature increases exponentially, so there is more and more research evidence to evaluate. With limited time to evaluate evidence, it is imperative that a busy clinician can access high-quality evidence. So we need to understand the levels and quality of evidence and ensure we use the most appropriate evidence to answer specific clinical questions.

Systematic assessments of research evidence are termed critical appraisal, which is 'the assessment of evidence by systematically reviewing its relevance, validity and results to specific situations' [4]. This is where the NICE Evidence online portal becomes important, as an assured way of quickly accessing trusted sources of such evidence beyond accredited guidelines.

Review of the chapters in this book

In this chapter, we wish to summarise what we have learned in the earlier chapters and relate this to the concepts of clinical quality, what it is, how to measure it and how to deliver the highest quality care. We also want to introduce the concept of quality improvement. Unfortunately, it is not true that breakthroughs in research quickly move into improved care for patients. Also it is not always the big research breakthrough that improves care, but more basic things such as the most appropriate person delivering the right care to the patients close to their home may really make the difference. So learning about service improvement will help us in our aspirations to translate what we learn about clinical quality and evidence into improved services.

What constitutes clinical quality and what is quality improvement?

Quality improvement is the duty of all health care professionals. To improve services requires us to bring together several themes. These are the development and use of evidence, and the reduction in variation by increasing development and implementation of guidance and audit. Other quality improvement techniques such as peer review, accreditation systems, confidential inquiry and systems from industry such as lean technology have an important role. In addition, the development of systems to enhance the ways teams work together and are led is vital. Finally, placing patients at the heart of our services, and ensuring we get regular patient feedback, is paramount to improving the safety of health care.

How does guidance support evidence-based medicine?

Chapter 1 discusses the history and rationale behind evidence-based medicine, and how this led to the use of guidance to control the issues generated by variability in research evidence. NICE's approach to developing robust clinical guidance uses clinicians and patients to review the best available evidence and generate sets of practical recommendations.

Linking evidence-based medicine to the development of guidance is vital, as the volume of evidence is so heavy that a practicing clinician would find it impossible to keep up with the evidence in isolation. Guidance needs to be used in a professional way, tailored to the individual patient, and with regard to the basic expertise of the clinician looking after patients [5]. With the team approach to the management of patients presenting acutely, doctors cannot expect to be experts in all or even many areas. So guidance is very useful in conferring safety information and will need to be tailored to the individual patient – see the example case study in Chapter 3.

When a clinician, whether it be hospital or in a primary care setting, is faced with a challenge of treating a patient with a complex medical problem, they may want to find clinical evidence to support appropriate treatment plans. They start by typing the subject matter into a leading popular search engine, which will bring up 100+ pages of information. It is impossible for the clinician to know which is accredited or not. Accredited guidelines appear at the top on NICE Evidence, however, and carry the NICE accreditation kite mark. This makes life much easier for the busy clinician.

Chapter 1 also reviews the challenges to implementation of guidance, including lack of clinical engagement and resource issues. Strategies are needed to aid implementation, and several approaches to this challenge have been taken from the service improvement work developed by industry. These vary from standard clinical audit to Plan, Do, Study, Act cycles, or PDSA for short (Figure 7.1).

But how does this work in practice? Consider a junior doctor managing an acute ward at night. He or she is handed over an elderly patient admitted following a fall in a care home. To the doctor, that patient appears well orientated and he has a good conversation when he takes over the ward. During the night, the doctor is called to the ward as the patient has become *confused*. What to do? The doctor can call for help but the senior cover might be very busy and the nurses very stretched. He or she can muddle through, or go to a nearby computer or tablet and type in www.evidence.org.uk and ask for information about delirium. Up will come the most recent, high-quality guidance and other trusted sources of evidence. So muddling through has been changed to a course of action based on the best possible evidence.

Chapter 3 explores the need for guidance in the world where we as clinicians are surrounded by evidence, but where we still need help to interpret and apply this evidence to treat the individual patient. Guidance helps, but we may feel bombarded by guidance from a range of different sources, and we therefore need to understand what constitutes good

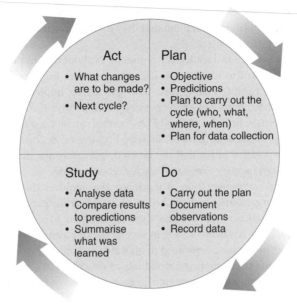

Fig. 7.1 Plan, Do Study, Act cycle.

guidance. NICE has recognised this need and has developed a system for accrediting those who produce guidance that follows international principles of guidance development. This chapter introduces the AGREE instrument (Appraisal of Guidelines Research and Evaluation), which is a tool for evaluating the quality of a guideline. NICE has taken this further by creating a system of accrediting makers of guidance, to streamline the process whereby clinicians can quickly access reputable evidence and guidance. Clinicians like nothing better than conflicting guidance. However, applying the AGREE tool allows us to assess the quality of the guideline and will help with its implementation.

What are the barriers to the use of guidance?

There are several very important chapters dealing with challenges in implementing guidance. There can be multiple reasons for these challenges, and the first of these may be 'we don't know what we don't know'. The drive to introduce and implement improvements in care may be because the relevant guidance recommendations have not been well publicised. Between clinicians, guideline producers, health care managers and patients, there should be enough personnel to address this area. Nevertheless, busy clinicians can be so consumed by looking after the patients in front of them that they do not have the time to reflect on improved treatments.

This is where clinical leadership comes in. Without this, improvements can be very hard to implement. Recruiting staff to the cause can best be done by clinical champions, who can drive implementation by informing those involved about possible changes and the rationale for improvements. Clinical audit and PDSA cycles can be used to check that improvements are taking place, thereby backing up such implementation. Other positive forces that can be used, but rarely are, include social media – often used by clinicians' use for other reasons.

Successful implementation of guidance also requires those who run health care organisations (the Board of a hospital or the partners of a primary care practice) to demonstrate their commitment to service improvement. Sadly this has been lacking in several of our recent service failures. The leaders of organisations need to allocate the implementation of such improvements to the named individuals as described in Chapter 2. The Board must routinely dedicate time to consideration of clinical effectiveness and ways of improving care.

NICE has a role in this also. They deploy a small number of local personnel who inform colleagues about recent developments at NICE and who promote and support the use of bespoke tools for assessing improvements in care. Finally, exploring alongside the NICE economic evaluations, what implementation can mean at a local level in terms of costs and savings expected from implementation.

Reflections on service improvement

Most health care systems have had quality improvement initiatives. Because clinical audit does not always have the desired impact, an additional approach has been suggested: 'Total Quality Management' (TQM) (among other names, including Six Sigma) that integrates quality, efficiency and leadership.

The major initiative is the PDSA cycle (Figure 7.1), which can be found in most service improvement plans. In fact, it was W. Edwards Deming who introduced the concept to the industry first. The principle is that when making changes to processes, it is safer and more effective to test out improvements on a small scale before implementing them across the Board. Using PDSA cycles enables you to test out changes before wholesale implementation and gives others, including patients, the opportunity to see if the proposed change will work.

Several examples would be as follows:

- Trying out a new way to make appointments for a general practitioner (GP) or a clinic.
- Trying out a new patient information sheet with a selected group of patients before introducing the change to all patient groups.

By building on the learning from these test cycles in a structured way, one can put a new idea in place with greater chances of success. As with any change, ownership is important to implementing the improvement successfully. If a range of colleagues is involved in trying something out on a small scale before it is fully operational, the barriers to change will be reduced. Ideas should only be implemented when all the alternatives have been considered and tested in all the possible ways.

How is clinical quality defined and how is it measured?

You can't improve that which you cannot measures

(Kenneth Kizer, Kaiser Permanente, USA,
Personal Communication)

Clinical quality is defined as the degree to which health services for individuals and populations increase the likelihood of desired health outcomes and are consistent with current professional knowledge. We think of quality in relation to three main dimensions (effectiveness, safety and patient experience), which can be integrated into three quality domains: structure, process and outcomes. These can be built into a grid such as Box 7.1, to give an overall picture of clinical quality.

This approach allows us to start to develop measures to assess the various components of clinical quality. Picking meaningful measures is crucial. An important principle to remember is that whatever we measure gets better, and this may be at the expense of that which is not measured. We tend to measure that which is easy to measure may not be that which is important. There are always negatives, so that we must look out for the unintended consequences of such measures.

These measures should preferably be the measures that are part of routine measurement and can be used to track change over time, and be used for benchmarking. Such metrics include clinical audit and other methods of assessing implementation of evidence and quality improvement. Measuring clinical quality requires a lot more than audit, although audit remains a very important component [6]. Using the findings of audit to improve services is, of course, the important next step.

Box 7.1 Quality illustrated through domains of structure, process and outcome

Quality dimensions	Clinically effective	Safe	Patient centred
Structure: Refers to the inherent characteristics that are associated with higher quality	1 A stroke ward 2 Primary care outreach nurse to elderly patients with long-term conditions 3 Systems and structures in place for setting standards and monitoring the quality of care 4 Procedure volumes 5 Advanced IT systems	1 Buildings with adequate clinical rooms with washing and air management systems 2 Staff with appropriate qualifications 3 Health and safety regulations understood	1 Systems and structures in place for monitoring patient experience 2 Systems in place to consult with patients 3 Systems in place to deal with complaints
Process	1 A primary care register compliant with • Cardiovascular (CV) disease guidance • diabetes guidance • childhood asthma 2 Are you compliant with evidence-based guidance, e.g. discharge from hospital following myocardial infection (MI) on appropriate medicines	1 Agreed guidance on hand washing 2 Plan around repeat prescriptions	1 Access to information 2 Confidentiality respected 3 Waiting times 4 Patient satisfaction training
Outcome	1 Reduced mortality following MI 2 Re-admissions following hospital admission 3 Survival rates following major surgery 4 Functional capacity following routine surgery	1 No of MRSA bacteraemias 2 Serious untoward events	1 Number of complaints 2 Patient satisfaction rates

Clinical audit

Some of the best information on quality improvement comes from clinical audit, both national audits and local audit. The reason is that, in general, it has clinical buy in with clinicians involved in designing what is measured as they understand what constitutes good and safe care. Obviously, we need patients, commissioners and managers involved in such decisions.

Clinical audit as a quality improvement process should involve members of a team working together to introduce best practice and make them routine, using quantitative feedback on the effects of change on process and outcomes.

There are many examples of excellent national audits and a host of local issues that need regular audit. All of these yield very valuable information.

How is a clinical audit performed?

As a health care worker, how would you go about performing an audit in a particular area? Firstly, and reiterating general advice already given in Chapter 4, one would want to talk to someone with expertise in the subject. Why not review the clinical audit programme in the institution where you work to see if the audit had already been performed or was about to be done. There might be a relevant national audit in existence and, if so, it would be useful to check their most recent learning points and whether there were any recommendations for local re-audits.

If a local audit is required, it is worth discussing the project in advance with the audit lead, and local clinicians and managers, as to be successful they will need to be involved and to support any resultant actions. Audits have to be done to standards or guidance, so it is imperative to seek these out. This should lead to an action plan with improvement at its heart, which needs to be widely promoted. Finally, arrangements will need to be made for re-audit following implementation of the changes.

In the general practice setting, clinical audit is crucial. Recently, a lot of work has been done on prescribing audits, so drugs that are over-prescribed and under-prescribed can be identified, and GPs are advised to review patients regularly who take a number of different medicines. In the coming years, a number of factors will affect prescribing and its associated spending, and it is difficult to forecast and quantify their long-term impact. These factors include new medicines, and cheaper versions of existing drugs are becoming available.

Whose responsibility is the achievement of high-quality care?

The development and implementation of guidance and standards with their associated audit need to be seen as mainstream in health care organisations. So those who lead such institutions, be it a highly prestigious large hospital or a small practice of clinicians, must have systems to assure themselves that the care they are providing is of high quality. This means that care is effective, safe and affords patients a good experience. The responsibility runs through an organisation from those who lead such organisations to those at the front line. Organisations must have direct lines of communication running through them allowing fast movement of such information. Those delivering care must be responsive to new and different ways of delivering care, which might not be what has traditionally been done.

There are ways of promoting such a culture and this comes down to leadership and having a highly trained and skilled workforce, open to innovation and change. Hopefully by implementing the measures outlined in this book, we will eliminate future serious failures and promote high-quality care.

Summary overview

Delivering high-quality care to patients is the responsibility of everyone who is involved in health care. To make this happen, we need comprehensive systems to disseminate evidence-based practice so all patients benefit from the best possible care. The most effective way of achieving this is to have systems supporting local clinicians to identify and understand best practice in their areas of expertise. There need to be systems of communication so that managers, including the Board, clinicians and patients are made aware of any changes. This can be supported by the use of guidance and audit to assure all that such implementation is taking place.

Learning from practice

1 The delivery of high-quality care is the responsibility of all working in health care and all who manage and deliver health care in all of its facets from the Board to front line.
2 Similarly, all need to understand that evidence is the cornerstone of delivery and they need to understand how to access such evidence either in the form of raw evidence or when condensed into guidance and standards.

3 Organisations must support their workforce in involving themselves in quality improvement by developing leadership skills so that all understand the roles of evidence, guidance, standards, metrics and audit and how to bring these together for the good of patients.

References

1 Walshe, K. and Shortell, S. (2004) When things go wrong: How healthcare organisations deal with major failures. *Health Affairs*, **23**, 103–111.
2 Steel, N., Bachmann, M., Maisey, S. *et al.* (2008) Self reported receipt of care consistent with 32 quality indicators: national population survey of adults aged 50 or more in England. *British Medical Journal*, **337**, a957.
3 Sackett, D., Rosenberg, W., Muir Grey, J. *et al* (1996) Evidence based medicine: what it is and what it isn't. *British Medical Journal*, **312**, 71.
4 Chambers, R. (1998) *Clinical Effectiveness Made Easy: First Thoughts on Clinical Governance*, Radcliffe Medical Press, Oxford.
5 Hampton, J. (2003) Guidelines – for the obedience of fools and the guidance of wise men? *Clinical Medicine*, **3**, 279.
6 Donabedian, A. (1966) Evaluating the quality of medical care. *The Milbank Memorial Fund Quarterly*, **44** (3pt 2), 166–203.

Further reading

Institute for Healthcare Improvement: http://www.ihi.org/Pages/default.aspx (accessed 10 April 2014).
Healthcare Quality Improvement Partnership: http://www.hqip.org.uk/ (accessed 10 April 2014).
Healthcare Improvement Scotland: http://www.healthcareimprovementscotland .org/welcome_to_healthcare_improvem.aspx (accessed 10 April 2014).
The Inquiry into the management of care of children receiving complex heart surgery at the Bristol Royal Infirmary: http://www.bristol-inquiry.org.uk/final_report /index.htm (accessed 10 April 2014).
The Mid Staffordshire NHS Foundation Trust Public Inquiry: http://www .midstaffspublicinquiry.com/report (accessed 10 April 2014).
Burgess, R. (ed) (2011) *Principles of Best Practice in Clinical Audit*, 2nd revised edition edn, Radcliffe Publishing Ltd, United Kingdom.
The King's Fund (2010) Getting the measure of quality, .. http://www.kingsfund .org.uk/publications/quality_measures.html (accessed 10 April 2014).
Department of Health (2008) *High Quality Care for All: NHS next stage review final report*, Department of Health, London.
Powell, A., Rushmer, R. and Davies, H. (2009) A systematic narrative review of quality improvement models in healthcare. Quality improvement Scotland. http://www .healthcareimprovementscotland.org/previous_resources/hta_report /a_systematic_narrative_review.aspx (accessed 10 April 2014).

Index

Achieving High Quality Care: Practical Experience from NICE, First Edition.
Edited by Gillian Leng, Val Moore and Sasha Abraham.
© 2014 John Wiley & Sons, Ltd. Published 2014 by John Wiley & Sons, Ltd.